ti O *Techniques in Orthopaedics*

Editorial Board

Techniques in Orthopaedics

Volume 4

Shoulder Surgery
in the Athlete

Edited by

Douglas W. Jackson, M.D.

Director
Southern California Center for Sports Medicine
Long Beach, California

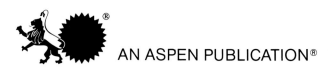 AN ASPEN PUBLICATION®

Aspen Systems Corporation
Rockville, Maryland
Royal Tunbridge Wells
1985

Aspen Systems Corporation
1600 Research Boulevard
Rockville, Maryland 20850

This publication was developed by University Park Press, Baltimore, Maryland.

ISBN 0-87189-257-X

Printed in the United States of America

1 2 3 4 5

Contents

Preface

Shoulder surgery in the athlete has seen an increasing success rate over the past ten years. This has been reflected both in scientific publications as well as the sports pages of our major newspapers. Athletes of all ages have come to expect more from the treating physician. No longer is the recommendation "give it up if it bothers you" as readily accepted by our patients. In addition to the high-level athlete that gets most of the attention in the press, the real shoulder problems confronting most physicians are seen in the aging recreational athlete. The aging athlete is part of the fastest growing portion of our population. More individuals today wish to continue to participate in racquet and throwing sports, swimming, and other activities that require strenuous repetitive use of the shoulder throughout their retirement years. These long-term demands and expectations on the shoulder have caused an increased interest in preserving shoulder function by being more aggressive in treating the younger patient and attempting to restore function where possible in our older population.

Advances in surgical treatment for a spectrum of shoulder problems are presented in this text by authors who have been contributors over a number of years and have a vast clinical experience in treating shoulder problems in the athlete. The chapters include some of the new concepts in glenohumeral instability, rotator cuff disease and impingement, intra-articular problems amenable to the arthroscope, and joint replacement. The results presented by these surgeons not only deal with the control of pain related to shoulder pathology but include expected restoration of function.

A further testimony to this expanding field and increasing expertise in shoulder surgery was the first open meeting of the American Shoulder and Elbow Surgeons, which was held in January 1985. Any time a scientific forum specifically dealing with an area develops, it only enhances our understanding of both the surgical and nonsurgical treatment of that particular joint. The shoulder will continue to be an area of rapid advancement over the next ten years. The chapters presented in this text should give the treating physician a basis for expanding and being part of this exciting new field.

The first chapter emphasizes the importance of the history, physical examination, and routine roentgenograms, which remain the basis of understanding and treating most shoulder problems in the athlete. There are a number of new diagnostic tests related to the shoulder such as contrast arthrograms, bursagrams, computed axial tomography, bone scans, electromyograms, and others, but none have replaced a carefully taken history or a meticulously carried out physical examination. However, the text points out that these new tests in select cases are often useful for integrating other findings into the diagnosis and management of the athlete with shoulder problems.

The anatomy and external landmarks of the shoulder have been well known to the orthopaedic surgeon operating on the shoulder. The arthroscope, during the past five years, has opened some new vistas and challenged some of our preconceived ideas on shoulder anatomy and function. Several chapters of this text are devoted to the appreciation of the arthroscopic shoulder anatomy and dynamics. The basis for the arthroscopic portals and approach to intra-articular pathology are reviewed in detail. The surgeon of the future will be doing more intra-articular arthroscopic surgical procedures for shoulder pathology. These procedures are going to continue to improve with better instrumentation in the next five to ten years.

The results of rotator cuff surgery and decompression of the coracoacromial arch have become more predictable, and the indications have been set forth in this text. The demands on the shoulder in the athletic population place the rotator cuff at risk and may contribute to its accelerated degeneration. The rotator cuff presents a spectrum of involvement from inflammation to impingement to partial tears to full-thickness tears. The surgical treatment needs to be selective and precise. Each of these categories represents a different challenge to the management of the athlete. Dr. Neer has shared his extensive experience in a series of active patients who have had prosthetic replacement; this is a field that is going to continue to expand in the future and is already giving quite good results in those carefully selected individuals. Glenohumeral arthritis, whether after dislocation or related to systemic disease, increasingly restricts the shoulder in the affected athlete.

Shoulder instability still must be clarified, particularly related to posterior instability, in the active and athletic patient and remains one of our continuing challenges in restoring shoulder function. The traditional surgical approaches for instability are presented and expected results are discussed. The new field of arthroscopic stabilization holds great promise but continues to be a procedure under extensive investigation. There are three aspects of controlling shoulder instability in the athlete: 1) controlling the symptomatic displacement, 2) attempting to minimize subsequent degenerative changes, and 3) avoiding restriction of motion to the point that it eliminates the desired shoulder function. The athlete needs motion and stability, which challenges the shoulder surgeon.

The contributors to this text have all confined themselves to the type of problems confronted by the physician treating the active and athletic patient with shoulder problems. They offer sound clinical judgment based on their present experience. The text will serve to update the physician about this new and changing field—shoulder surgery in the athlete.

DWJ

Contributors

James R. Andrews, M.D.
Clinical Assistant Professor
Section of Sports Medicine
Dept. of Orthopaedic Surgery
Tulane University School of Medicine;
Director of Orthopaedic Training
Hughston Orthopaedic Clinic, P.A.
6262 Hamilton Road
Columbus, Georgia 31995

John J. Brems, M.D.
Fellow, Shoulder and Elbow Surgery
New York Orthopaedic Hospital at Columbia-
  Presbyterian Medical Center
161 Fort Washington Avenue
New York, New York 10032;
Cleveland Clinic
9500 Euclid Avenue
Cleveland, Ohio 44106

William G. Carson, Jr., M.D.
Assistant Clinical Professor of Orthopaedics
University of South Florida
Tampa Orthopaedic Clinic
602 South Howard Avenue
Tampa, Florida 33606

Richard B. Caspari, M.D.
Tuckahoe Orthopaedic Associates, Ltd.
Tuckahoe Medical Center
8919 Three Chopt Road
Richmond, Virginia 23229

James M. Colville, M.D.
San Jose Medical Group
Orthopaedic and Podiatry Dept.
45 South 17th Street
San Jose, California 95112

Jay S. Cox, M.D.
Sports Medicine Consultant
U.S. Naval Academy
2 Wood Road
Annapolis, Maryland 21402

Andrew R. Einhorn, R.P.T., A.T.C.
Assistant Director of Physical Therapy
Southern California Center for Sports Medicine
2760 Atlantic Avenue
Long Beach, California 90806

Ben K. Graf, M.D.
Knee and Sports Medicine Fellow
Memorial Medical Center
Long Beach, California 90806

Thomas J. Harries
Lcdr., M.C., U.S.N.
Director of Sports Medicine
U.S. Naval Academy
2 Wood Road
Annapolis, Maryland 21402

Richard J. Hawkins, M.D.
Clinical Associate Professor
St. Joseph's Hospital
University of Western Ontario
450 Central Ave.
Suite 107
London, Ontario N6B 2E8
Canada

Douglas W. Jackson, M.D.
Director, Southern California Center for
   Sports Medicine
2760 Atlantic Avenue
Long Beach, California 90806

Frank W. Jobe, M.D.
Southwestern Orthopaedic Medical Group
501 E. Hardy Street
Inglewood, California 90301

Benjamin Ling, M.D.
Biomechanics Laboratory
Centinela Hospital Medical Center
Inglewood, California 90301

Leslie S. Matthews, M.D.
Assistant Professor, Orthopaedic Surgery
Johns Hopkins Hospital;
Assistant Chief of Orthopaedic Surgery
Union Memorial Hospital
Baltimore, Maryland 21218

Gary W. Misamore, M.D.
Clinical Assistant Professor
Indiana University
Indianapolis, Indiana 46260

Charles S. Neer, II, M.D.
Professor, Clinical Orthopaedic Surgery
Columbia University College of Physicians and
   Surgeons at Columbia-Presbyterian Medical
   Center
161 Fort Washington Avenue
New York, New York 10032

Paul R. Reiman, M.D.
Knee and Sports Medicine Fellow
Memorial Medical Center
Long Beach, California 90806

Russell F. Warren, M.D.
Associate Professor of Orthopaedic Surgery
Cornell University Medical College;
Director, Sports Medicine Service
Hospital for Special Surgery
535 E. 70th Street
New York, New York 10021

Allan Murray Wiley, M.Ch., F.R.C.S.
Associate Professor (Orthopaedics)
University of Toronto
Suite 101
25 Leonard Avenue
Toronto, Ontario M5T 2R2
Canada

Bertram Zarins, M.D.
Assistant Clinical Professor of Orthopaedic
   Surgery
Harvard Medical School;
Chief, Sports Medicine Unit
Massachusetts General Hospital
15 Parkman Street—Level 4
Boston, Massachusetts 02114

tiO *Techniques in Orthopaedics*

Diagnosis of the Painful Athletic Shoulder

1

Douglas W. Jackson
Paul R. Reiman

Active individuals who use their shoulders repetitively and strenuously and develop a disabling pain pattern can be a diagnostic challenge to the physician. Over the past decade physicians have gained greater insight into the different diagnostic entities and mechanisms of injury that can cause shoulder disability in this population. While a variety of new diagnostic techniques have contributed to this increased understanding, the history and physical examination remain the mainstays in the diagnosis and in the decision-making process for treatment and rehabilitation. An accurate diagnosis requires a thorough understanding of the functional anatomy of the region; the biomechanics of the throwing, racquet, or swimming motions; and the common pathological syndromes that occur in the region.

Functional Anatomy

The shoulder girdle includes four joints or articulations: the glenohumeral joint, the acromioclavicular joint, the sternoclavicular joint, and the scapulothoracic articulation. It is the glenohumeral joint and the associated soft tissue problems that will be emphasized in this text, but their interrelations with the other supporting structures remain important. The glenohumeral joint has a ball-and-socket configuration with a large arc of motion. There is a normal range of arm elevation in either flexion or abduction of 160 degrees in men and 175 degrees in women. This arc is obtained not only by glenohumeral motion, but also through scapulothoracic motion. According to Perry (23), this approximates a 2:1 ratio but does have a wide variation. The glenohumeral joint itself is a relatively unstable joint when

1

one considers only the bony structures, as the glenoid fossa of the scapula is very shallow. The anterior stability is enhanced by the glenoid fossa being retroverted approximately 7 degrees and the humeral head retroverted 30 degrees (31). The stability is enhanced greatly by the surrounding soft tissue structures. The glenoid labrum is a fibrous structure, triangular in cross section, which increases the surface area of humeral head coverage. This coverage increases from approximately 25–30% of the humeral head with the glenoid fossa alone to 65–75% by adding the labrum (23). However, this varies considerably. Another soft tissue structure that enhances glenohumeral stability is the capsule, which attaches circumferentially about the glenoid and the anatomical neck. Due to the large range of motion of the gleno-humeral joint, the capsule is redundant in certain areas, depending upon the position of the arm. The superior capsule is lax when overhead elevation is performed, and the inferior capsule has a redundant fold when the arm is at the side. The capsule is reinforced anteriorly by the superior, middle, and inferior glenohumeral liga-ments (31). It has been shown by Saha (27) that these glenohumeral ligaments are the prime restraints against dislocations of the humeral head by external rotation and abduction. The inferior glenohumeral ligament has been reported to be of *considerable* importance in both the symptoms and surgical treatment of instabil-ities of the shoulder in the athletic population. Another supporting structure of the glenohumeral joint is the musculotendinous cuff unit, comprised of the subscapu-laris anteriorly, the supraspinatus superiorly, and the infraspinatus and teres minor posteriorly. The contribution of these different musculotendinous units and gle-nohumeral ligaments to the stability of the glenohumeral joint varies with the arm's position (31).

The glenohumeral joint functions under the coracoacromial ligament, which is a vestigial, thick, fibrous structure contributing to the roof of the glenohumeral joint. Directly superior to the glenohumeral joint are the undersurfaces of the acromioclavicular joint and the acromion. The differentiating pathology in the acromioclavicular joint, the rotator cuff tendons, and the subdeltoid bursa can sometimes be difficult.

The biceps tendon passes intra-articularly from the bicipital groove across the superior portion of the humeral head and then attaches directly on to the glenoid labrum and the neck of the glenoid. The function and contributions of this tendon are being appreciated more and more, particularly with the advent of shoulder arthroscopy. The relationship of the biceps tendon to the glenoid labrum and its role as a depressor of the humeral head and decelerator of the forearm are of increasing interest in the active person involved in throwing sports.

Biomechanics

The motions required for the athletic shoulder are best evaluated in the throwing athlete and the swimmer. The act of throwing is generally divided into three phases: cocking, acceleration and follow-through (23). During the cocking phase the hu-merus is abducted and externally rotated. This motion has been divided by Jobe et al. (10, 11) and Jobe and Jobe (8) into an early phase and a late phase. The deltoid begins to show marked activity during the early cocking phase, when the shoulder is held at approximately 90 degrees of abduction. Towards the end of this early phase, when external rotation begins, the supraspinatus, infraspinatus, and teres minor are activated, with the supraspinatus showing the greatest activity. At the end of the cocking phase, these rotator cuff muscles become less active and the subscapularis begins to fire to decelerate the external rotation of the glenohumeral joint. During the acceleration phase the triceps musculature exhibits considerable activity, as do the pectoralis major and latissimus dorsi. The serratus anterior also is extremely active during this acceleration phase. The final phase is the follow-through, which begins after ball release through the cessation of motion. The musculature most active during this phase is the subscapularis, which is internally rotating the shoulder. The remainder of the rotator cuff and the deltoid fire towards the end of the follow-through to decelerate the arm, with the pectoralis major and the latissimus dorsi activated to a lesser degree (10, 11).

The biomechanics of shoulder motion of other major sports are surprisingly similar to that of the thrower. In tennis, the forehand stroke and serve demonstrate very similar mechanics, and in the backhand stroke the mechanics are reversed. In the backhand stroke the shoulder is forcefully externally rotated and abducted, as opposed to internally rotated and adducted in the thrower or in the forehand tennis stroke. The swimmer also shows a similar motion whether the stroke is free style, butterfly, or breast stroke. The major contractile forces in the pull-through phase again show the arm internally rotating and adducting. Then the arm externally rotates and abducts to place the arm once again in a position for a power stroke. These phases of shoulder motion are important to recognize because most overuse and malalignment syndromes can be directly correlated to the muscular activities in these specific phases (23, 25).

History

The historical information the athlete gives regarding his shoulder pain is extremely important and usually provides more information than either the physical exam or any specific diagnostic test. The physical examination and diagnostic tests usually confirm the suspicions engendered by the history. As with any musculoskeletal problem, the patient should be asked to describe the presenting and any past symptoms, their duration, character, and relation to other activities (9, 12). The patient's daily activities and athletic requirements should be determined. Often the patient's participation in a specific competitive athletic event is not the only factor aggravating the shoulder.

The complete past medical history is particularly important in the older recreational athlete who may have underlying systemic disease or other contributing factors. A history of previous trauma, surgery, or symptoms in the area should be elicited. Neck pathology, cardiac disease, referred abdominal dysfunction, and possible malignancy may occasionally present as a shoulder disability or restriction. An appropriate neurological and vascular history of the neck, thoracic outlet, and upper extremity is essential to rule out referred pain or symptoms. This referred pain to the shoulder is uncommon but should not be overlooked in the active individual.

The effect of the patient's pain on his or her athletic performance is probably the most important facet of the history, and an attempt to correlate the pain with the different phases of the aggravating motion is often helpful. Does the pain only present in a particular phase of shoulder motion? The patient's attempt to reproduce the pain by placing the arm in the exact position of dysfunction is also a very important diagnostic clue (25, 33). Does the pain only occur during the athletic activity, or does it continue through the night? Night pain can be indicative of not only the more classically recognized neoplastic conditions, but also of an acute inflammatory process of the tendons and bursas about the shoulder. These more common inflammatory processes of the shoulder may present with rather severe, continuous pain when compared to a tendonitis or bursitis in another portion of the body (15).

At the completion of the history, in the athletic population, shoulder problems usually fall into one of three major categories: the acute (sudden onset) injury, the overuse syndrome, or the underlying biomechanical malalignment abnormalities that can be aggravated by repetitive use. Of course, there can be a great deal of overlap between these three categories. The acute and chronic problems may overlap or occur in the same shoulder.

Physical Examination

The examination should begin when the patient walks into the examining room. The shirt or blouse should be removed for the shoulder examination with provisions made for the proper gowning of all female patients so as not to impede or hinder the examination. It is mandatory that both shoulders be available for the examination. Inspection of the shoulder usually includes looking for atrophy of the supraspinatus, infraspinatus, or deltoid musculature. Muscular atrophy of the triceps, biceps, and brachialis musculature should be documented. Any gross deformities of the thorax, scapula, neck, or upper extremity should be noted. Acromioclavicular separation with its concurrent swelling and deformity can usually be seen. It is important to note any previous surgical or traumatic scars about either the shoulder, neck, or upper arm. In the highly competitive athlete, there is often hypertrophy in the musculature in the dominant arm when compared to the nondominant arm.

Palpation of the bony and soft tissue structures about the shoulder should be done systematically and gently to reduce any patient anxiety. Initial palpation should be performed over both shoulders with the cupped hand to determine any increased warmth in the symptomatic shoulder. Palpation should include the sternoclavicular joint and the entire length of the clavicle laterally to the acromioclavicular joint, noting any protuberance, crepitus, or tenderness. The acromioclavicular joint should be palpated with both arms at rest and while the patient flexes, extends, and adducts his shoulder (8).

The acromion can be followed around to the spine of the scapula, noting any tenderness along the spine. The inferior and medial borders of the scapula should also be palpated, both with the arm at rest and in motion, moving from flexion and extension to help delineate winging of the scapula or the "snapping scapula syndrome" (18). The coracoid process is identified and palpated. Finally, attention should be paid directly to the head of the humerus and the adjacent soft tissue. The greater tuberosity and the bicipital groove are palpated. The biceps tendon, when palpated bilaterally, is normally somewhat tender to palpation, and it is the difference in this tenderness that is the important diagnostic clue. Direct tenderness over the muscle bellies of the pectoralis, supraspinatus, infraspinatus, deltoid, biceps, and triceps should be documented and may be indicative of cervical radiculopathy or brachial plexus radiculopathy or neuropathy. The rotator cuff can be palpated throughout its course by flexing and extending the shoulder to selectively bring out the anterior and posterior portions of the supraspinatus tendon from underneath the acromion (19).

Cervical spine pathology with referred pain to the shoulder is more frequent in the age 40 and older group. Restrictions in cervical motion and compressing the head to reproduce the symptoms are noted. The brachial plexus neuropathies are more common in the younger contact athlete. Percussion over the potential location of suprascapular nerve entrapment should be performed.

The neurological examination includes the upper extremity reflexes and sensory examination of the cervical and thoracic dermatomes. Older patients with suspected referred pain from the cervical area should have their lower extremity reflexes checked, looking for signs of clonus. The Adson Test may be helpful in giving insight into the occasional thoracic outlet syndrome. Palpation should be performed in the cervical, supraclavicular axillary areas for signs of lymphadenopathy.

Testing and documentation of the patient's range of motion of the glenohumeral joint includes abduction, adduction, extension, flexion, internal rotation, and external rotation. Two quick screening tests, combining all of these motions, are to have the patient put his hand behind his head, which involves the external rotators and abductors, followed by the motion of putting the hands behind the lumbar spine area, which involves extension, internal rotation, and abduction. The highest level they can reach of their thoracic spinous process with their thumb can be documented. The individual planes of motion should then be isolated as much as possible to help further delineate the pathology. Overhead extension should be checked, ideally in the supine position, with comparison between the shoulders. It is important to note the degree and point of onset of scapulothoracic motion during abduction. This should begin at approximately 90 degrees of abduction. Any crepitation, popping, snapping, or any subjective feelings that the patient exhibits when these range-of-motion tests are performed may be helpful (9). The athlete should be asked to simulate the motion involved in his or her sport in an attempt to reproduce the symptomatology.

Manual muscle testing is an important part of the examination. The patient should be observed closely, not only for specific muscle weakness which can sometimes be very subtle, but also for any pain that is elicited by this specific testing. Testing should include resisted internal and external rotation of the shoulder with the arm at the patient's side and the elbow flexed to 90 degrees (Figures 1–1 and 1–2). The supraspinatus muscle tendon unit may be isolated by having the patient place his arm in a position of 90 degrees forward flexion, 30 degrees abduction, and maximal internal rotation of the entire arm with the little finger up in the "tea cup position" (Figure 1–3). Signs of impingement syndrome can be elicited by forcing the humeral head into the undersurface of the acromion, either by forced elevation or by flexing the arm 90 degrees and forcefully adducting and internally rotating the glenohumeral joint (7, 22, 33) (Figure 1–4).

Bicipital tendon pathology may be elicited by the Yergason test in which the patient has his elbow flexed 90 degrees and the examiner applies an external rotation force to the humerus and attempts to extend the elbow. The bicipital tendon may also be directly palpated by internally and externally rotating the shoulder in 90 degrees of abduction (20) (Figure 1–5).

Instability of the shoulder can sometimes be a very subtle finding with the instability occurring in many directions (4, 6, 8, 16, 21, 24, 26, 28, 32). Initially, with the arm resting at the patient's side, anterior and posterior translation as well as superior and inferior translation of the humerus in the glenoid fossa can be tested on both the symptomatic and asymptomatic shoulder. Any clicks or snaps as well as abnormal translation should be noted. The shoulder apprehension test can be performed with the patient in the prone position with the arm hanging over the edge of the table, or with the patient in the standing or sitting position (Figure 1–6). The arm should then be very gently abducted and externally rotated in a slow, deliberate fashion with a force producing anterior subluxation. The more unstable shoulder may produce the apprehension sign in the patient. Posterior subluxation is more difficult to interpret but can be produced by placing a very small amount of pressure in the axilla while forward flexing and extending the arm. A certain amount of posterior translation may be normal for that patient. The

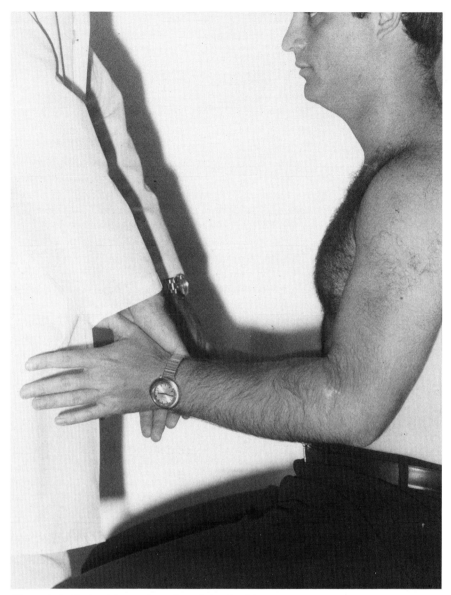

Figure 1–1 Resisted internal rotation of the shoulder.

uninvolved shoulder can often be used as the standard. Always ask the patient if they can voluntarily sublux their shoulder. This may be helpful in assessing the patient with subluxation.

It is sometimes helpful to have the athletic fatigue his shoulder by performing aggravating motion followed by a repeat examination. This will sometimes help the diagnosis to become more evident in a difficult shoulder problem (25).

Radiographic Examination

Radiographic examination of the athletic shoulder should be tailored to the results of the history and physical examination so that maximum information can be attained with minimal radiographic exposure. The routine radiographic examination, using anteroposterior projections in varying degrees of rotation, with and without

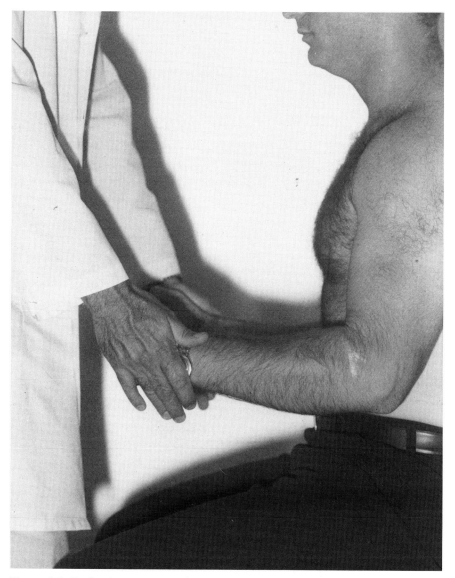

Figure 1–2 Resisted external rotation of the shoulder.

stress, can be helpful to discern large lesions of the humeral head, gross instability, and, to some degree, acromioclavicular pathology (5, 14) (Figure 1–7). However, it is very poor for demonstrating rotator cuff or glenoid labrum pathology. Several additional views have been shown to be helpful to further delineate that pathology. The axillary West Point projection is used to bring the anteroinferior aspect of the glenoid rim into focus. The view is taken posterior to anterior with the patient in the prone position and the arm extended. The West Point view may demonstrate irregularities or ossification along the anterior and inferior rim of the glenoid in patients with recurrent anterior subluxation or dislocation of the shoulder (33) (Figures 1–8 and 1–9). Another view that may be helpful is the scapula-Y or lateral scapula view, which places the scapula in the form of the Y with the coracoid anterior, the acromion posterior, and the glenoid in the center. The relationship of the humeral head to the glenoid fossa is then evaluated. There are several modifications of these views that may be helpful to or preferred by certain examiners. Whatever routine is used, at least two views in different planes are needed.

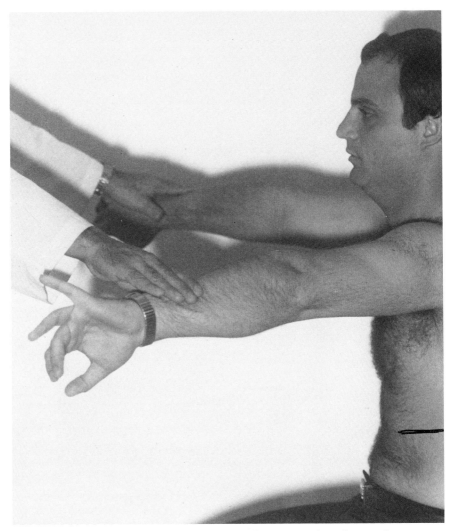

Figure 1–3 Testing for dysfunction of the supraspinatus musculotendinous unit.

Arthrography of the shoulder joint has been, in the past, a very helpful test to document full thickness rotator cuff tears. However, it is a very poor quantitative test, not delineating the size of the tear in the rotator cuff or reflecting partial tears. To correct these deficits, a multitude of other techniques including double contrast arthrography and bursography have been combined with either tomography or computed tomography and have been found to be helpful in evaluating certain rotator cuff tears and the status of the glenoid labrum (1–3, 8, 13, 17, 29) (Figure 1–10). Subacromial bursography has been suggested to be helpful in predicting the surgical results in those patients with impingement syndrome (30) and intact rotator cuffs.

When there is a high index of suspicion of nerve involvement, either due to direct trauma, traction, compression, or inflammation, an electromyelogram may be indicated. It may not show significant changes for 2–3 weeks following an acute injury. This is sometimes very helpful in delineating the "dead arm syndrome" of the thrower, which can be suggestive of either instability or a neuropraxia. The electromyelogram is also helpful in evaluating atrophy and weakness where there is a question as to the underlying etiology.

A relatively new and potentially helpful tool is arthroscopy. The techniques of diagnostic and operative shoulder arthroscopy have progressed rapidly over the

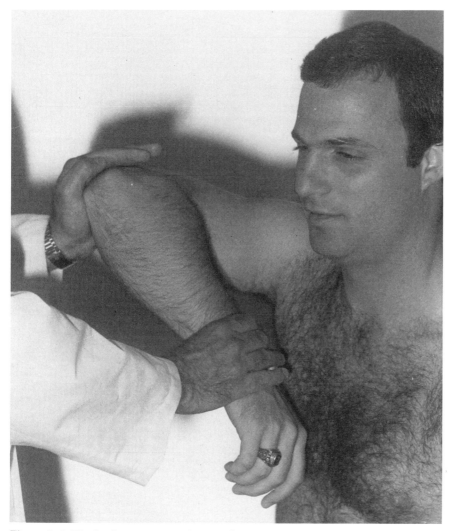

Figure 1–4 The impingement test. (See text for detailed description.)

past several years. Arthroscopy is particularly helpful in delineating lesions in the glenoid labrum, the intra-articular portion of the biceps tendon, the glenohumeral ligaments, and the undersurface of the rotator cuff. It has not been as helpful in full-thickness tears of the rotator cuff, impingement pathology, or other extra-articular conditions of the athletic shoulder. However, the application of the arthroscope will increase as instrumentation and techniques improve. Careful scrutiny of this increasing experience is warranted.

Conclusion

More specific diagnosis and treatment of shoulder problems of the athlete challenge a new and rapidly expanding field within orthopaedics and sports medicine. Yet with the advent of new techniques and treatments, one must not neglect the essential history and physical examination, which continues to provide us with the greatest amount of information. Necessary for each athlete is an individual diagnosis, with his or her own goals, motivation, and specific sport skill level all being very important considerations in the patient's care plan.

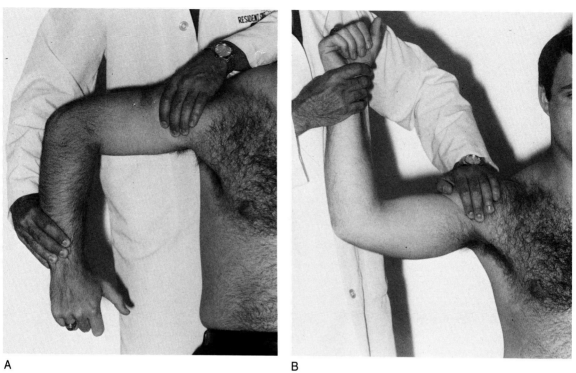

A   B

Figure 1–5, A and B Testing for instability and dysfunction of the biceps tendon (long head).

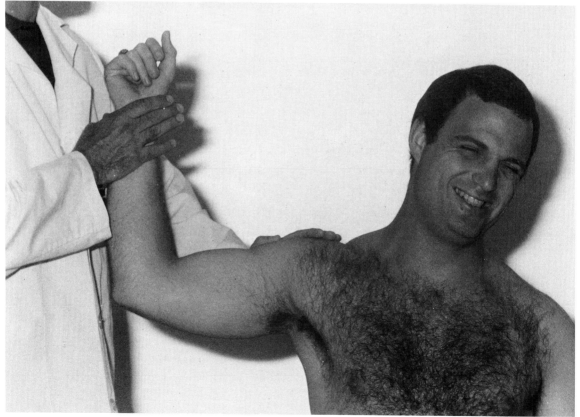

Figure 1–6 Testing for anterior instability of the shoulder. (A positive apprehension sign is shown.)

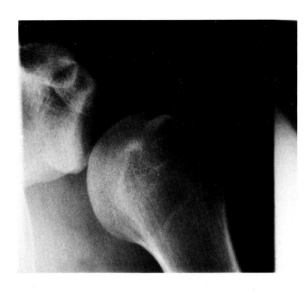

Figure 1–7 Inferior instability of the glenohumeral joint shown in a pole vaulter by applying traction to the arm. The opposite shoulder did not show this translation.

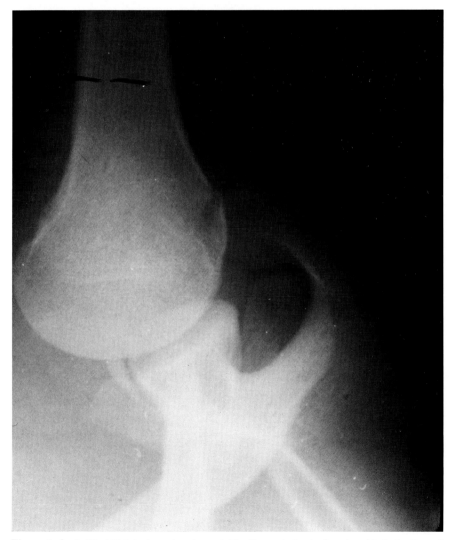

Figure 1–8 A West Point view showing calcification anterior to the glenoid, indicative of anterior capsular injury.

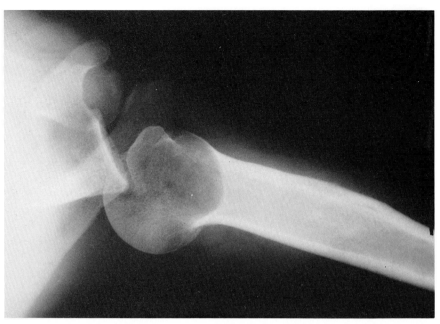

Figure 1–9 An axillary view showing a posteriorly dislocated humeral head with a large reverse Hill-Sachs lesion.

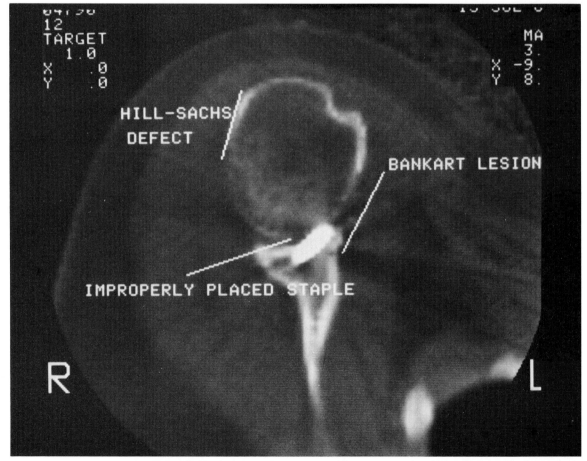

Figure 1–10 A computed tomogram without contrast showing an improperly placed staple within the glenohumeral joint.

References

1. Berman JL, Shaub MS. Arthrography of the shoulder. Clinics in Sports Medicine 2:291–308, 1983
2. Braunstein EM, O'Connor G. Double contrast arthrography of the shoulder. J [Am] Bone Joint Surg 64:192–195, 1982
3. Danzig L, Resnick D, Greenway G. Evaluation of unstable shoulders by computerized tomography. Am J Sports Med 10:138–141, 1982
4. Foster CR. Multidirectional instability of the shoulder in the athlete. Clinics in Sports Medicine 2:355–368, 1983
5. Hansen NM. Epiphyseal changes in the proximal humerus of an adolescent baseball pitcher. Am J Sports Med 10:380–384, 1982
6. Hastings DE, Coughlin LP. Recurrent subluxation of the glenohumeral joint. Am J Sports Med 9:352–355, 1981
7. Hawkins RJ, Habeika PE. Impingement syndrome in the athletic shoulder. Clin Sports Med 2:391–405, 1983
8. Jobe CW, Jobe FW. Painful athletic injuries of the shoulder. Clin Orthop 173:117–124, 1983
9. Jobe FW, Moynes DR. Delineation of diagnostic criteria and rehabilitation programs for rotator cuff injuries. Am J Sports Med 10:336–339, 1982
10. Jobe FW, Moynes DR, Tibone, JE, Perry J. An EMG analysis of the shoulder in pitching. Am J Sports Med 12:218–220, 1984
11. Jobe FW, Tibone JE, Perry J, Moynes DR. An EMG analysis of the shoulder in throwing and pitching. Am J Sports Med 11:3–5, 1983
12. Leach RE, Schepsis AA. Shoulder pain. Clinics in Sports Medicine 2:123–135, 1983
13. Kilcoyne RF, Matson FA. Rotator cuff tear measurement by pneumotomography. AJR 140:315–318, 1983
14. Kohler R, Trilland, JM. Fracture and fracture separation of the proximal humerus in children. J Pediatr Orthop 3:326–332, 1983
15. MacNab I. The Painful Shoulder. Sound slide presentation, American Academy of Orthopaedic Surgeons, Chicago, 1965
16. Matsen FA, Zuckerman JD. Anterior glenohumeral instability. Clinics in Sports Medicine 2:319–338, 1983
17. McGlynn FJ, El-Khoury G, Albright JP. Arthrotomography of the glenoid labrum in shoulder instability. J Bone Joint Surg [Am] 64:506–518, 1982
18. Neviaser RJ. Painful conditions affecting the shoulder. Clin Orthop 173:63–69, 1983
19. Neviaser RJ, Neviaser TJ. Lesions of the Musculotendinous Cuff of the Shoulder: Diagnosis and Management. In: American Academy of Orthopaedic Surgeons. Instructional Course Lectures, vol 30, pp 239–273. AAOS, Chicago, 1981
20. O'Donoghue D. Subluxating biceps tendon in the athlete. Clin Orthop 164:26–29, 1982
21. Pappas AM, Goss TP, Kleinman PK. Symptomatic shoulder instability due to lesions of the glenoid labrum. Am J Sports Med 11:279–288, 1983
22. Penny JM, Welsh RP. Shoulder impingement syndromes in the athlete and their surgical management. Am J Sports Med 9:11–15, 1981
23. Perry J. Anatomy and biomechanics of the shoulder in throwing, swimming, gymnastics and tennis. Clinics in Sports Medicine 2:247–270, 1983
24. Protzman RR. Anterior instability of the shoulder. J Bone Joint Surg [Am] 62:909–918, 1980
25. Richardson AB. Overuse syndromes in baseball, tennis, gymnastics and swimming. Clinics in Sports Medicine 2:379–390, 1983
26. Rowe CR, Zarins B: Recurrent transient subluxation of the shoulder. J Bone Joint Surg [Am] 63:863–872, 1981
27. Saha AK. Mechanics of elevation of the glenohumeral joint. Acta Orthop Scand 44:668–678, 1983
28. Samilson RL, Prieto V. Posterior dislocation of the shoulder in athletes. Clinics in Sports Medicine 2:369–378, 1983
29. Shuman WP, Kilcoyne RF, Matson FA, et al. Double contrast computed tomography of the glenoid labrum. AJR 141:581–584, 1983

30. Strizak AM, Danzig L, Jackson DW, et al. Subacromial bursography: An anatomical and clinical study. J Bone Joint Surg [Am] 64:196–201, 1982

31. Turkel SJ, Panio MW, Marshall JL, Girgis FG. Stabilizing mechanisms preventing anterior dislocations of the glenohumeral joint. J Bone Joint Surg [Am] 63:1208–1217, 1981

32. Warren RF. Subluxation of the shoulder in athletes. Clinics in Sports Medicine 2:339–354, 1983

33. Yocum LA. Assessing the shoulder: History, physical examination, differential diagnosis, and special tests. Clinics in Sports Medicine 2:281–289, 1983

Anatomy and Portals for Arthroscopic Surgery of the Shoulder

2

Richard B. Caspari

Arthroscopy of the shoulder was introduced to this country as far back as 1972 (7). Recently, however, shoulder arthroscopy has become a more common procedure. Concomitantly, the techniques for doing this procedure have become more sophisticated, and the types of procedures that can be performed are increasing rapidly. Diagnostic arthroscopy of the shoulder has increased our understanding of the pathophysiology of several maladies of the shoulder. Direct observation of labral tears has led to the conclusion that several etiologies may be responsible for this entity (3). Labral tears may not only be associated with instability but may be traumatic, associated with the throwing motion, or be degenerative in nature (2). Observations regarding instabilities of the shoulder have also been reported, including detachment of the labrum, as in the Bankart lesion; fraying of the labrum secondary to anterior translocation of the humeral head on the glenoid; subtle articular Hill-Sachs lesions; and incompetence of the anteroinferior glenohumeral ligament (6). The rather common incidence of partial rotator cuff tears has been reported to be associated with short-term good results from debridement (1). In addition, synovectomy, removal of loose bodies, and chondroplasty have been introduced as arthroscopic techniques. Perhaps one of the most exciting prospects is that of repair of shoulder instability, and these techniques are presently being clinically investigated by the author and by L.L. Johnson (personal communication).

As with any surgical procedure, an excellent understanding of anatomy in all planes is necessary to accomplish arthroscopic surgery of the shoulder. This article then will review the gross and arthroscopic anatomy of the shoulder as related to the techniques of establishing the various portals for arthroscopic surgery of the shoulder (5). The uses of each portal will also be described.

External Anatomy

Knowledge of the external anatomy and the relationships of the palpable landmarks of the shoulder are the key to accurate portal placement. Unlike the knee, the shoulder is surrounded by a rather thick soft tissue envelope, which makes the accurate placement of portals somewhat difficult. Once a portal is established, it should be maintained at all times as it is fairly difficult to reintroduce an instrument or cannula exactly through the same hole in the soft tissue. Multiple passages of instruments in and out of the shoulder will lead to rather massive soft tissue insufflation with saline, resulting in the inability to perform the procedure as planned.

The palpable landmarks about the shoulder incude the clavicle and coracoid anteriorly, the acromion laterally, and the scapular spine posteriorly. These structures are, for the most part, subcutaneous and can be palpated in the most muscular or obese of individuals (Figure 2–1). The acromioclavicular joint anteriorly marks the junction of the anterior and lateral aspects of the shoulder, just below which the coracoid can be palpated. The deltoid is a rather large, thick muscle encompassing the shoulder from anterior to posterior and prevents any direct palpation of the rotator cuff, humeral head, or tuberosities of the shoulder. The biceps tendon anteriorly may be palpated, however, by rolling it under one's finger as it enters the bicipital groove. Posteriorly the scapular spine is palpated as a ridge beginning at the posterior point of the acromion and extending medially for the entire width of the scapula. This ridge divides the supraspinatus and infraspinatus fossae and is one of the keys for placement of both the posterior and superior portals.

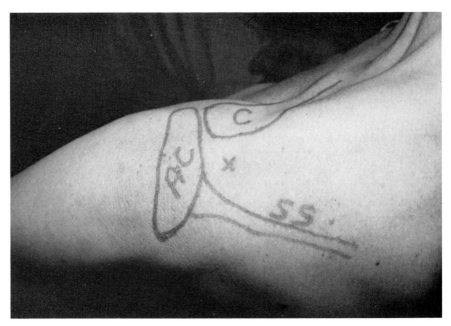

Figure 2–1 Bony landmarks for arthroscopy of the shoulder can be easily palpated.

Anatomy and Portal Placement

Posterior Portal

The posterior approach is the most common portal used for arthroscopy of the shoulder. It allows visualization of most of the intra-articular structures. The external landmark for establishment of this portal is the posterior point of the acromion, which is the junction of the acromion and the scapular spine. The location of the portal is approximately one thumb's breadth or 2 cm inferior to this point (Figure 2–2). The coracoid process is palpated anteriorly and the angle of entry is from the point of portal placement to the coracoid. Prior to placement of the arthroscopic cannula, the shoulder may be entered with a spinal needle and insufflated with saline. Some surgeons prefer to place the cannula directly into the shoulder without preinsufflation. As the cannula is placed into the shoulder with a sharp trocar, passage through the fascia of the deltoid can be palpated, and upon entry of the cannula into the shoulder joint, a distinct "pop" can be felt. A blunt trocar should then be utilized for final placement of the cannulas in the shoulder. The cannula traverses several structures on entry into the joint. The skin and subcutaneous tissue have been lacerated with a no. 11 blade, and the posterior thickness of the deltoid is then pierced. The subdeltoid bursa usually extends this far posteriorly and both walls are traversed. The cannula then passes through the muscular belly of the infraspinatus or, in some cases, in the interval between the

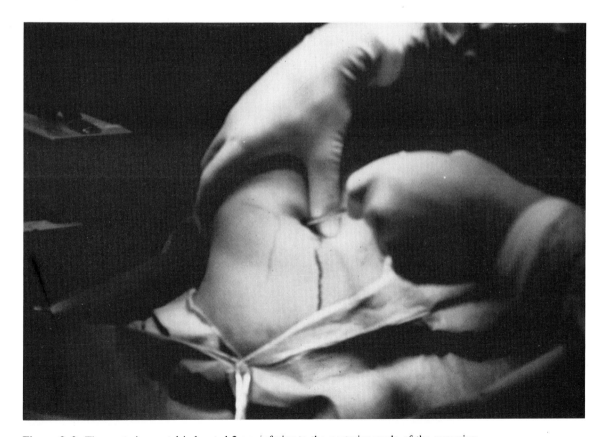

Figure 2–2 The posterior portal is located 2 cm inferior to the posterior angle of the acromion.

infraspinatus and teres minor (Figure 2–3). Finally the capsule and synovium are pierced, allowing entry into the glenohumeral joint.

This entry is quite safe, passing below the acromion and through the inferior muscle belly of the infraspinatus, near its interval with the teres minor. The areas of concern are the quadrangular and triangular spaces that respectively transmit the posterior humeral circumflex artery and axillary nerve, and the scapular circumflex artery to the posterior aspect of the shoulder. The quadrangular space is defined inferiorly by the teres major, laterally by the humerus, medially by the long head of the triceps, and superiorly by the teres minor, which provides the margin of safety for the posterior portal to avoid injury to the neurovascular structures. The triangular space is medial to the long head of the triceps. Innervation of the infraspinatus is supplied by the suprascapular nerve as it passes from the supraspinatus fossa to the infraspinatus fossa around the scapular spine. The teres minor receives its innervation from a branch of the axillary nerve as it passes beneath its lower border. Thus the innervation of these two muscles is not endangered by the posterior portal.

The posterior portal is used primarily as an arthroscopic portal and allows almost complete visualization of the glenohumeral joint. The most consistent landmark is the biceps tendon as it passes through the joint, arising from the superior portion of the glenoid labrum and exiting the joint through the bicipital tendon sheath (Figure 2–4). The tendon may be visualized and followed throughout its intra-articular course. The humeral head can be visualized almost entirely, beginning superiorly at the greater tuberosity, extending inferiorly to the axilla, and including the entire posterior portion of the humeral head. Greater visualization can be obtained by manipulation of the shoulder and rotation of the humerus throughout its range of motion. The very anterior aspect of the humeral head is not visualized from the posterior approach. However, the entirety of the glenoid may be examined quite nicely from this approach. The glenoid faces slightly anterior and has a bean-shaped configuration with an indentation in its anterior mar-

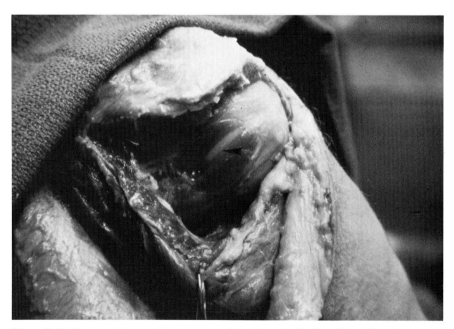

Figure 2–3 The posterior portal passes approximately at the border of the infraspinatus and teres minor muscle bellies.

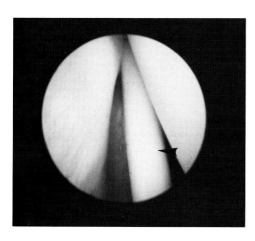

Figure 2–4 The biceps tendon is the most consistent intra-articular landmark for arthroscopy of the shoulder.

gin. The normal glenoid labrum is seen to be closely adherent to the glenoid circumferentially. The labrum is quite thick at its attachment to the glenoid neck, tapering to a rather thin margin that extends slightly over the face of the glenoid. The labrum also provides for the insertion of several structures into the glenoid neck. The biceps tendon achieves its origin via the superior labrum, and the anterior glenohumeral ligaments achieve their attachment through the labrum anteriorly. Three glenohumeral ligaments have been described: they are the superior, middle, and inferior glenohumeral ligaments. These ligaments represent thickenings in the anterior capsule, and the superior and middle glenohumeral ligaments are inconsistent in their presence. The inferior glenohumeral ligament, however, is a rather large structure that is consistently present and is viewed quite nicely when the shoulder is brought into abduction and external rotation. In this position the ligament is seen anteriorly as a large band that provides a buttress to prevent anterior translocation of the humeral head on the glenoid. The other most prominent structure seen in the area of the anterior capsule is the tendon of the subscapularis muscle. When dissected anatomically, the tendon of the subscapularis appears as a rather broad and flat structure. Arthroscopically, however, the tendon appears rounded and somewhat smaller than the biceps tendon. This portion of the subscapularis tendon, which is visible from the interior of the joint, is the superior border of the tendon which is, indeed, thickened and rounded on anatomical dissection (Figure 2–5). At the most medial extent of this tendon and just above it, one may encounter what appears to be a hole in the anterior capsule. This represents an intra-articular communication with the subscapular bursa or recess, which lies between the subscapularis muscle and the neck of the scapula. Inferiorly, the entirety of the axillary space can be examined, with the capsule seen to be attached to the inferior neck of the glenoid and the shaft of the humerus. Occasionally, loose bodies will gravitate to this area. Superiorly, the rotator cuff can be further examined. The supraspinatus tendon is seen to form the roof of the shoulder and attach to the greater tuberosity. By angling the scope the superior portion of the infraspinatus can also be seen; however, the entirety of the infraspinatus and teres minor tendons cannot be visualized from this portal.

In some cases the subdeltoid bursa may also be examined utilizing the posterior approach. If the bursa has been chronically inflamed, the walls will be relatively thick, allowing insufflation with saline and entrance with an arthroscope. However, if the bursa is normal, attempted entry with the arthroscope will simply tear the filmy wall and prohibit insufflation. The roof of the subdeltoid bursa is

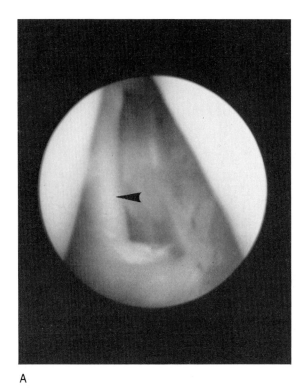

A

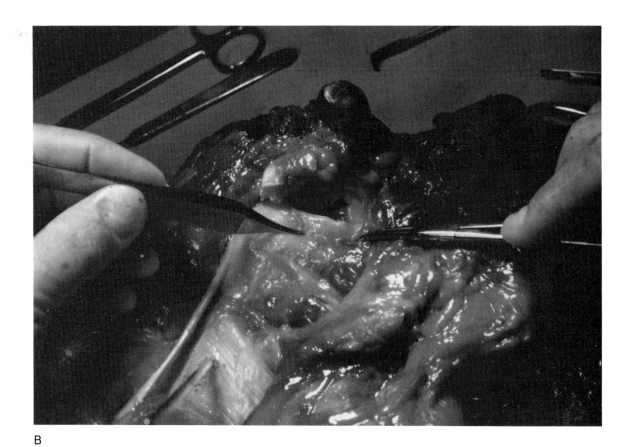

B

Figure 2–5 Arthroscopic (**A**) and anatomical (**B**) appearance of the superior margin of the subscapularis tendon.

represented by the rotator cuff, which can be visualized by internally and externally rotating the shoulder and thus parading the cuff in front of the arthroscope. The acromioclavicular joint and the coracoacromial ligament, however, are not visualized through the bursa.

Anterior Portal

The anterior portal is most commonly used to pass instrumentation into the joint. It may be established directly by passing a spinal needle from the anterior and visualizing its entrance into the joint. Once a satisfactory angle is established, the puncture wound is made anteriorly and a cannula is directed into the joint. This method is somewhat difficult in that the soft tissue envelope of the shoulder anteriorly is quite thick, making this direct method somewhat inconsistent and difficult to attain. The preferred method is to pass the arthroscope from the posterior portal to the point on the anterior capsule at which entry is desired. This generally lies within the triangular space bounded superiorly by the biceps tendon, inferiorly by the subscapularis tendon, and medially by the anterosuperior portion of the glenoid. The tip of the arthroscope is placed against the capsule in this area and the arthroscope is removed from its sheath. A Steinmann pin is passed through the sheath of the arthroscope, puncturing the capsule and appearing through the skin on the anterior aspect of the shoulder. The puncture wound is then made around the pin. The pin and arthroscope sheath are carefully retracted and the arthroscope is reinserted into its sheath. The blunt end of the Steinmann pin can then be visualized within the joint. A cannula is passed over the Steinmann pin into the shoulder joint and the pin is removed. Once the portal has been established, it should never be lost, and if the cannula is to be removed for any reason, a pin should be placed through the cannula and left in its place to preserve the tract.

Anteriorly the portal should be lateral to the coracoid process, which can be palpated through the muscle belly of the deltoid and is the primary landmark to avoid injury to the neurovascular structures on the anterior aspect of the shoulder. The conjoined tendon inserts on the coracoid, and some 3 cm inferior to the process, and along the medial border of the conjoined tendon lies the musculocutaneous nerve. Any placement of the portal medial to the coracoid process places this nerve in jeopardy (Figure 2–6).

The portal is used primarily for instrumentation and allows access intra-articularly to the biceps tendon, the superior portion of the rotator cuff, and the entire anterior portion of the labrum. Posteriorly, the labrum may be reached in its superior portion but not inferiorly. The entire anterior glenoid neck and face of the glenoid also are instrumented via this portal. The humeral head can be reached, except posteriorly. The posterior recess behind the posterior lip of the glenoid is also inaccessible from this portal.

Supraspinatus Fossa Portal

The supraspinatus fossa portal is most commonly used as an inflow portal (4). Inflow may also be accomplished by establishing a second portal anteriorly or posteriorly; however, this results in crowding both the inside and outside of the joint. The supraspinatus fossa portal may also be utilized for visualization and instrumentation; however, it is limited, as manipulation of the arthroscope or instrument is inhibited by the bony structures surrounding the portal.

The point of entry is in the supraspinatus fossa, which may be palpated by the index finger and is a soft spot bordered anteriorly by the posterior margin of

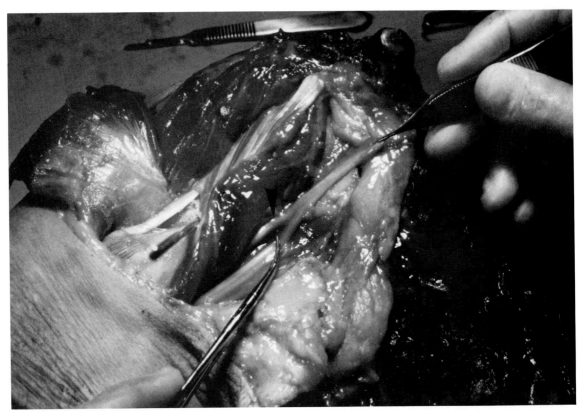

Figure 2–6 The anterior portal is lateral to the coracoid process to avoid injury to the musculocutaneous nerve on the medial side of the conjoined tendon.

the clavicle, laterally by the medial border of the acromion, and inferiorly by the scapular spine. The portal is established by passing a spinal needle through this soft spot at a 30-degree angle from the horizontal and in a slightly posterior direction. The needle should appear in the shoulder joint above the superoposterior portion of the glenoid neck. A puncture wound is then made, and a cannula is passed into the joint along the same tract and is tucked into the posterior recess, out of the way of the arthroscope and instrumentation being passed from the other portals.

The supraspinatus fossa is covered by the trapezius muscle. Underneath the trapezius the supraspinatus muscle belly fills the entirety of the supraspinatus fossa, from which it takes its origin. The supraspinatus muscle then passes underneath the acromion, where it becomes tendonous and forms the superior portion of the rotator cuff. The portal of entry passes through the muscle belly portion of the supraspinatus and causes no injury to the rotator cuff (Figure 2–7). The supraspinatus receives its innervation via the suprascapular nerve that enters the fossa via the suprascapular notch. The notch divides the scapula into a medial two-thirds and lateral one-third. The suprascapular nerve and vessel pass along the floor of the supraspinatus fossa, supplying the muscle, and exit the fossa around the most lateral aspect of the scapular spine. On anatomical dissection the nerve and vessel are seen to lie approximately 3 cm medial to the suprascapular portal (Figure 2–7). As the cannula passes through the supraspinatus muscle belly, it pierces the shoulder capsule just superior to the neck of the glenoid. The attachment of the biceps is anterior to this point of entry.

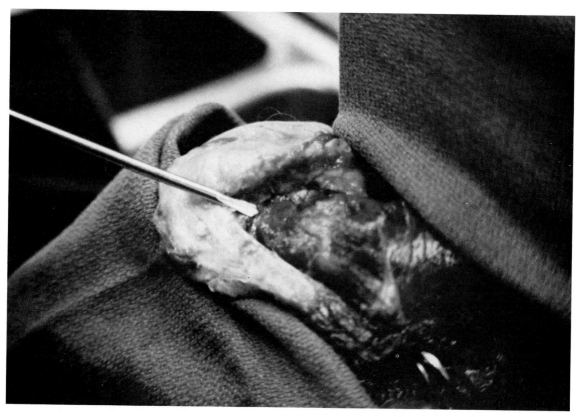

A

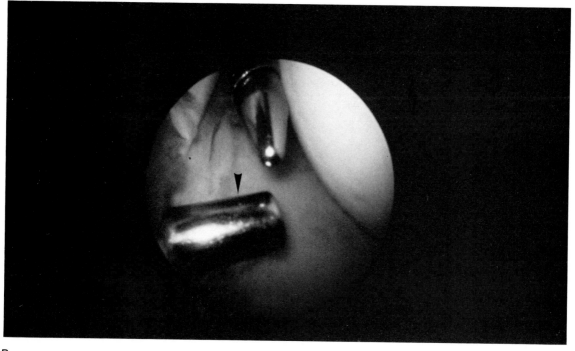

B

Figure 2–7 The cannula passes through the muscle belly of supraspinatus (**A**) and enters the shoulder superior to the neck of the glenoid (**B**).

When used as an arthroscopic portal, the superior neck of the glenoid and the entire posterior labrum and posterior recess are well visualized. Also, the posterior aspect of the humeral head may be examined. The anterior aspect of the shoulder cannot be well visualized via this portal because manipulation of the scope is tethered by the bony confines of the portal. Similarly, instrumentation passed through this portal is hampered.

Summary

Three basic portals for arthroscopic surgery of the shoulder have been presented. A precise knowledge of the anatomy associated with these portals and the anatomical relationships, both inside and outside of the joint, is necessary to accomplish successful procedures arthroscopically. We continue to learn more about the shoulder from arthroscopic investigations and more sophisticated procedures continue to be introduced. In the long run, this should result in more successful procedures and decreased morbidity for our patients.

References

1. Andrews JR, Broussard T, Carson WG. Arthroscopy of the shoulder in the management of partial tears of the rotator cuff: A preliminary report. Journal of Arthroscopic Surgery (to be published)
2. Andrews JR, Carson WG. The arthroscopic treatment of glenoid labrum tears in the throwing athlete. Orthop Trans 8:44, 1984
3. Caspari RB. Shoulder arthroscopy: A review of the present state of the art. Contemp Orthop 4:523–30, 1982
4. Caspari RB, Whipple TL, Meyers JF. The Neviaser portal for shoulder arthroscopy. Paper presented at the Annual Meeting of the Arthroscopy Association of North America, New Orleans, 1984
5. Hollinshead, WH. Textbook of Anatomy. Harper & Row, New York, 1962
6. McGlynn FJ, Caspari RB. Arthroscopic findings in the subluxating shoulder. Clin Orthop 183:173–178, 1984
7. Wiley AM, Older MWJ. Shoulder arthroscopy: Investigations with a fiber optic instrument. Am J Sports Med 8:31–33, 1980

Arthroscopic Anatomy of the Shoulder

3

James R. Andrews
William G. Carson, Jr.

Arthroscopy has become firmly established as a diagnostic and therapeutic modality in the knee joint. Its use for the evaluation of a shoulder joint is also becoming more firmly established (1–6, 10, 11, 17–20, 27). To be effective, arthroscopy of the shoulder needs to be performed in a systematic and reproducible fashion. In addition, a knowledge of the normal and normal variational arthroscopic anatomy of the shoulder is a prerequisite for those performing this procedure.

This chapter is devoted to the description of the normal anatomy of the shoulder as viewed arthroscopically. The majority of the anatomical structures are viewed through the posterior portal, using the technique described by the senior author (1–5).

To ensure a thorough and reproducible arthroscopic examination of the shoulder, the following structures should be identified in sequential order: the biceps tendon; the humeral head; the glenoid; the glenoid labrum; the superior, middle, and inferior glenohumeral ligaments; the subscapularis tendon and recess; and the rotator cuff.

Anatomical Structures

Biceps Tendon

The biceps tendon is the first structure to be identified after entering the shoulder joint and is the key to maintaining proper orientation during the arthroscopic examination. With the patient in the lateral decubitus position and the shoul-

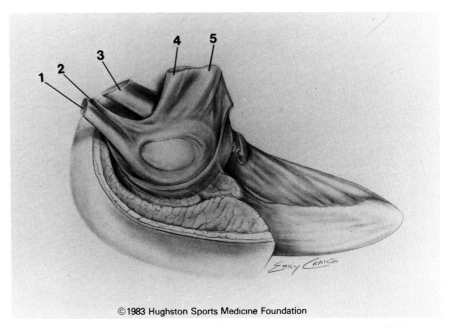

Figure 3–1 Arthroscopic anatomy of a right shoulder with the arm abducted 70 degrees. The major structures of the anterosuperior capsule are 1) tendon, long head of the biceps; 2) superior glenohumeral ligament; 3) subscapularis tendon; 4) middle glenohumeral ligament; 5) inferior glenohumeral ligament.

der in 70 degrees of abduction and 15 degrees of forward flexion, the biceps tendon is oriented approximately 10–15 degrees away from an imaginary vertical line (Figure 3–1). The biceps tendon attaches to the supraglenoid tubercle at the posterosuperior aspect of the glenoid rim and is intimately related to the glenoid labrum in this area (Figure 3–1). Externally rotate the patient's arm to facilitate visualization of the biceps tendon. Many times the biceps tendon can be followed anteriorly to the bicipital groove. Its surface should appear smooth, glistening, and free of any adhesions, partial tears, or fraying.

Humeral Head and Glenoid

Once the biceps tendon is inspected and proper orientation to the anatomy is regained, examine the articular surfaces of the humeral head (superiorly) and the glenoid (inferiorly). With the patient in the lateral decubitus position, one can examine approximately one-third of the articular surface of the humeral head, which is oriented in 30 degrees of retroversion. Examine the entire articular surface by rotating the arthroscope superiorly and rotating the humeral head into internal and external rotation. The glenoid cavity can also be examined arthroscopically. It is a pear-shaped cavity approximately one-fourth the size of the humeral head. Note the attachment of the biceps tendon to the posterosuperior aspect of the glenoid rim for orientation to the exact area of the glenoid being examined.

Glenoid Labrum

The glenoid labrum is a wedge-shaped structure that borders the glenoid cavity and provides inherent stability to the glenohumeral joint and restricts anterior and posterior excursion of the humerus (7, 14). Controversy exists as to the exact composition of the glenoid labrum. It has been described as consisting of hyaline cartilage, fibrocartilage, and fibrous tissue (7, 9, 15, 20, 21, 22). The glenoid surface of the labrum is continuous with the hyaline cartilage of the glenoid cavity while the capsular surface blends with the joint capsule.

The glenoid labrum should appear smooth and should lack fraying, partial tearing, or hypermobility. Begin the inspection at the insertion of the biceps tendon through the superior portion of the labrum into the supraglenoid tubercle and then continue anteriorly and inferiorly. Occasionally, additional distraction of the arm is required to examine the inferior rim of the glenoid labrum. As the arthroscope is retracted and posteriorly rotated, inspect the posterior rim of the glenoid labrum. Inspection of the posterior aspect of the glenoid may also be performed by placing the arthroscope anteriorly and viewing the posterior aspect of the labrum from this approach.

Glenohumeral Ligaments

The superior, middle, and inferior glenohumeral ligaments (Figures 3–1 and 3–2) are thickenings of the anterior capsule of the shoulder and stabilize the anterior and inferior portions of the joint capsule (8, 9, 20, 22–24). When viewed arthroscopically the glenohumeral ligaments are anteriorly displaced due to the fluid distension within the shoulder joint. In actuality these ligaments lie closer to the glenoid labrum. On occasion the glenohumeral ligaments will be seen to have distinct labral origins rather than their usual capsular origins.

The superior glenohumeral ligament, together with the coracohumeral ligament, stabilizes the shoulder when the arm is in the adducted, dependent position (8, 20). The ligament has two proximal attachments: one to the superior aspect of

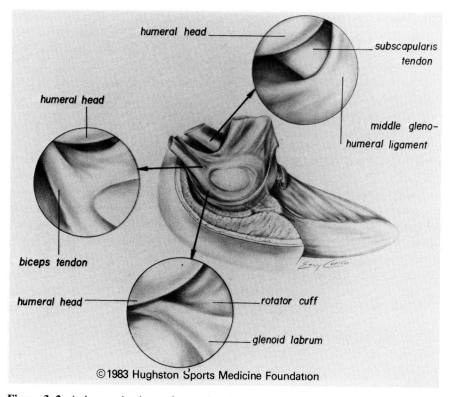

©1983 Hughston Sports Medicine Foundation

Figure 3–2 Arthroscopic views of normal anatomy.

the labrum, conjoined with the biceps tendon, and one to the base of the coracoid (24). The superior glenohumeral ligament courses laterally to insert on the anterior aspect of the anatomical neck of the humerus. This ligament usually can be seen near the insertion of the biceps tendon into the superior aspect of the glenoid; however, on occasion it is hidden behind the biceps tendon and may appear to be absent.

The middle glenohumeral ligament stabilizes the shoulder joint when the shoulder is abducted to 45 degrees (24). Although the attachments of this ligament are quite wide, they may be difficult to visualize arthroscopically. However, the middle portion of the middle glenohumeral ligament can usually be seen just posterior to the subscapularis tendon, with which it sometimes fuses. The ligament extends from just beneath the superior glenohumeral ligament along the anterior border of the glenoid to the junction of the middle and inferior one-third of the glenoid rim. It appears to blend with the anterior capsule and inserts near the lesser tuberosity over the anterior aspect of the anatomical neck of the humerus.

The inferior glenohumeral ligament has been shown to stabilize the glenohumeral joint when the arm is abducted to approximately 90 degrees (24). This triangular ligament arises from the anteroinferior margin of the labrum and inserts into the inferior aspect of the surgical neck of the humerus. It usually can be viewed arthroscopically when the arm is in the abducted position, thus tightening this ligament. Distraction of the arm may be required to place the arthroscope entirely across the glenohumeral joint to view the region of the axillary recess and thus the area of the inferior glenohumeral ligament.

Subscapularis Tendon and Recess

With the arm in the abducted position, one can visualize the posterosuperior edge of the subscapularis tendon in the anterior aspect of the shoulder between the superior and middle glenohumeral ligaments (Figure 3–1). The subscapularis tendon occasionally may be obscured by, or appear to blend with, the middle glenohumeral ligament. The subscapularis recess can be found over the anterior aspect of the shoulder directly beneath the subscapularis tendon in the region of the middle glenohumeral ligament.

Rotator Cuff

The arthroscopic examination of the rotator cuff begins by identifying the biceps tendon to obtain proper orientation. The supraspinatus portion of the rotator cuff can be seen just superior to the biceps tendon. Rotate the arthroscope superiorly and slightly toward the humeral head to facilitate visualization. Slight posterior retraction of the arthroscope will reveal the insertion of the tendinous portion of the rotator cuff into the humeral head. The infraspinatus and teres minor portions of the rotator cuff can be seen by directing the arthroscope posteriorly and superiorly.

Discussion

Arthroscopic examination of the shoulder must be performed in a methodical fashion to ensure accuracy. The surgical technique described by the authors (1–5) has been most successful in realizing these goals. We have found that a 4-mm, 30-degree-angled arthroscope allows optimum visualization of the shoulder joint. Using the biceps tendon as an internal landmark, examine each anatomical structure in sequential order, as follows: the biceps tendon, the humeral head and glenoid, the glenoid labrum, the glenohumeral ligaments, subscapularis tendon and recess, and the tendons of the rotator cuff.

Much variation in the glenohumeral ligaments has been described (9, 12–14, 16, 20, 23, 26) and may be a source of confusion when viewing the anterior capsular structures arthroscopically. Mosely and Overgaard (20) found that the inferior glenohumeral ligament was the most consistent of the glenohumeral ligaments in their series of patients, as did Turkel et al. (24), who described a thick "superior band" and a smaller "axillary pouch" portion of the inferior glenohumeral ligament. DePalma et al. (13, 14), however, found the superior glenohumeral ligament to be consistently the most well defined in their cadaveric specimens, whereas the inferior glenohumeral ligament was ill-defined or absent in 44%. In the DePalma group's specimens, the middle glenohumeral ligament was well defined in 71% and absent or ill-defined in the remaining 29%.

The variable relationship of the glenohumeral ligaments can result in variations in the subscapularis recess and occasionally can obscure the subscapularis tendon. The subscapularis recess may be found superior or inferior to the middle glenohumeral ligament or both. Occasionally, the absence of a middle glenohumeral ligament can result in a single large subscapularis recess (14). Care should be taken not to misinterpret these normal anatomical variations as pathological lesions in the anterior capsule of the shoulder.

Conclusion

For arthroscopy of the shoulder to be effective, the examination requires attention to detail and execution in a systematic fashion. When the appropriate surgical technique is performed with adequate distraction to the glenohumeral joint (1–5), all of the intra-articular structures may be visualized quite readily. The long head of the biceps tendon is used as a landmark for proper orientation when viewing the intra-articular structures. A knowledge of the normal arthroscopic anatomy of the shoulder, as well as the normal variational anatomy, is essential for the arthroscopic examination to be successful. Using the proper technique and identifying the intra-articular structures in sequential order should produce a thorough, systematic arthroscopic examination of the shoulder.

References

1. Andrews JR, Broussard T, Carson WG. Arthroscopy of the shoulder in the management of partial tears of the rotator cuff: A preliminary report. Arthroscopy (to be published)
2. Andrews JR, Carson WG. Shoulder joint arthroscopy. Orthopedics 6:1157–1162, 1983
3. Andrews JR, Carson WG. The arthroscopic treatment of glenoid labrum tears in the throwing athlete. Orthop Trans 8:44, 1984
4. Andrews JR, Carson WG, Hughston JC. Arthroscopic surgery of the shoulder. Orthop Trans 5:499, 1983
5. Andrews JR, Carson WG, Ortega K. Arthroscopy of the shoulder: Technique and normal anatomy. Am J Sports Med 12:1–7, 1984
6. Andrews JR, Hughston JC, Carson WG, Holford D. Arthroscopy of the shoulder. Orthopaedics Today 3:11, Nov 1983
7. Bankart ASB. The pathology and treatment of recurrent dislocation of the shoulder joint. Br J Surg 26:23–29, 1938
8. Basmajian JV, Bazant FJ. Factors preventing downward dislocation of the abducted shoulder. J Bone Joint Surg [Am] 41:1182–1186, 1959

9. Bost FC, Inman VT. The pathological changes in recurrent dislocation of the shoulder. A report of Bankart's operative procedure. J Bone Joint Surg [Am] 24:595–613, 1942

10. Carson WG, McLeod WD, Andrews JR. An analysis of the long head of the biceps tendon in relation to glenoid labrum tears. Am J Sports Med (to be published)

11. Caspari RB. Shoulder arthroscopy: A review of the present state of the art. Contemp Orthop 4:523–530, 1982

12. DePalma AF. Degenerative lesions of the shoulder joint at various age groups which are compatible with good function. In: American Academy of Orthopaedic Surgeons. Instructional Course Lectures, vol. 7, pp 168–180. AAOS, Chicago, 1950

13. DePalma AF. Surgery of the shoulder. JB Lippincott, Philadelphia, 1973

14. DePalma AF, Callery G, Bennett GA. Variational anatomy and degenerative lesions of the shoulder joint. In: American Academy of Orthopaedic Surgeons. Instructional Course Lectures, vol 6, pp 255–280. AAOS, Chicago, 1949

15. Dutoit GT, Roux D. Recurrent dislocation of the shoulder. A twenty-four year study of the Johannesburg stapling operation. J Bone Joint Surg [Am] 38:1–12, 1956

16. Flood V. Discovery of a new ligament of the shoulder joint. Lancet 1:672–673, 1829

17. Johnson LL. Arthroscopy of the shoulder. Orthop Clin North Am 11:197–204, 1980

18. Johnson LL. Diagnostic and Surgical Arthroscopy, pp 376–389. CV Mosby, St. Louis, 1981

19. Lombardo SJ. Arthroscopy of the shoulder. Clinics in Sports Medicine 2:309–318, 1983

20. Mosely JF, Overgaard. The anterior capsular mechanism in recurrent anterior dislocation of the shoulder. J Bone Joint Surg [Br] 44:913–927, 1962

21. Rowe CR, Patell D, Southmayd WW. The Bankart procedure: A long-term, end-results study. J Bone Joint Surg [Am] 60:1–6, 1978

22. Rowe DR, Zarins B. Recurrent transient subluxation of the shoulder. J Bone Joint Surg [Am] 63:863–872, 1981

23. Schlemm F. Ueber die Verstarkungsbander am Schultergelenk. Archiv für Anatomic und Physiologie 45–48, 1853

24. Turkel SJ, Panio MW, Marshall JL, et al. Stabilizing mechanism preventing anterior dislocation of the glenohumeral joint. J Bone Joint Surg [Am] 63:1208–1217, 1981

25. Warwick R, Williams P (eds). Gray's Anatomy of the Human Body, 35th ed. WB Saunders, Philadelphia, 1973

26. Weitbrecht J. Syndesmology, or A Description of the Ligaments of the Human Body. (EB Kaplan, trans). WB Saunders, Philadelphia, 1969

27. Wiley AM, Older MB. Shoulder arthroscopy. Investigation with a fibro-optic instrument. Am J Sports Med 8:31–38, 1980

Evaluation and Treatment of Glenoid Labrum Tears

4

Bertram Zarins
Leslie S. Matthews

In this chapter we will discuss glenoid labrum injuries. We will review the anatomy of the labrum, mechanisms of labrum injury, and establishing the diagnosis of a torn labrum. We will discuss special techniques that can be useful in confirming pathology of the labrum, including the role of arthroscopy. Finally, we will present our methods of treatment of labrum injuries.

Historical Perspective

The evolution of our current understanding of the glenoid labrum in relation to shoulder injuries can be traced through three phases. The first deals with the recognition of injury to the labrum in recurrent anterior dislocations of the shoulder, as described by Bankart and Cantab (3) and popularized by Rowe et al. (21). Blazina and Satzman (4), Protzman (18), Rowe and Zarins (22), and others ushered in the second phase with descriptions of similar injuries in shoulders that sustained recurrent subluxations. Most recently, Pappas et al. (17), Andrews et al. (2), and others (6, 11) have demonstrated that tears of the labrum can occur in stable shoulders, especially in throwing athletes.

Early studies on the glenoid labrum were performed by clinicians interested in defining the pathology in recurrent glenohumeral dislocations. Bankart and Cantab (3) referred to the labrum as the "fibrocartilagenous glenoid ligament" and felt that the common cause of recurrent anterior instability of the shoulder was "shearing of the fibrous capsule" from the "fibrocartilagenous glenoid ligament." They stated that spontaneous healing of this lesion was infrequent.

Townley (23) thought that tearing of the labrum could occur as the result of the capsular separation or be secondary to the direct contact of the humeral head against the labrum as the head came out of the socket. He was the first to imply that pathology of the labrum itself did not lead to glenohumeral instability. Townley stated that ''the labrum has little if any role in prevention of dislocation.'' He emphasized the importance of capsular disruption as the basic pathology in instability.

Moseley and Overgaard (15) analyzed in detail the gross, histological, and functional anatomy of the glenoid labrum. Based on histological examination, they suggested that the labrum was predominantly fibrous and not fibrocartilagenous tissue. They believed that the shape of the labrum changed with shoulder rotation. With medial rotation, a ''washer shaped functional labrum'' was noted that ''straightened out and disappeared'' with lateral rotation. Rowe et al. (21) refined the understanding of the role of the labrum in shoulder stability and outlined treatment based on the pathology.

Blazina and Satzman (4) in 1969 ushered in the second phase when they described recurrent transient subluxation of the shoulder. In their series, 66% of patients were found at surgery to have labral pathology. Rowe and Zarins (22) in 1981 described the ''dead arm syndrome'' related to throwing or other overhead activities and described the ''apprehension test.'' In their series, 64% of the patients operated upon were noted to have labral pathology. In only one-half of these patients was the subluxation recognized by the patients themselves or their referring physicians. Rockwood (19) provided a classification of the various types of subluxation.

Recent reports have described injury of the labrum in shoulders of throwing athletes in which no instability could be recognized. Pappas et al. (17) documented 16 cases in which symptomatic tears of the glenoid labrum were not associated with ''instability.'' In these throwing athletes, resection of the torn labral tissue alone relieved symptoms. Andrews and Carson (1) reported similar cases in which shoulder symptoms were relieved by arthroscopic resection of torn labral tissue.

Anatomy

The glenoid labrum is a fibrocartilaginous structure that is located at the circumference of the glenoid cavity and serves to ''deepen'' the glenoid cavity. More importantly, the labrum is intimately associated with the shoulder capsule, and, in fact, serves to anchor the casule to the glenoid rim. The labrum is a thicker and stronger structure in areas where the capsule is also thicker, such as anteriorly and anteroinferiorly, and thinner and weaker in areas of thinner capsule, such as posterosuperiorly. When viewed in cross section, the labrum can be seen to blend with the articular cartilage of the glenoid cavity on one side and with the scapular neck on the other.

From the standpoint of glenohumeral stability, the labrum becomes important because it serves as the attachment point of the capsule. Turkel et al. (24), in sequential cutting studies, demonstrated that the inferior glenohumeral ligament is the main stabilizing structure of the anterior aspect of the shoulder when the arm is abducted. The inferior glenohumeral ligament blends with the anterior labrum as they attach to the anterior glenoid rim (Figure 4–1). ''Detachment'' of the anterior labrum can result in a loss of integrity of the major anterior stabilizing tissue of the shoulder and result in instability. The superior and middle glenohumeral ligaments can also attach to the labrum, but variability is more common in the anatomy of these structures (8).

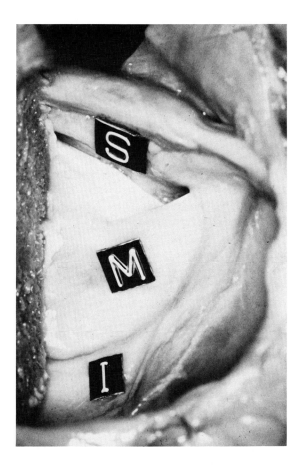

Figure 4–1 Gross anatomical specimen, posterior view, left shoulder with humeral head removed. The relationship of the anterior capsular ligaments to the glenoid labrum is shown: S, superior; M, middle; and I, inferior glenohumeral ligaments. The superior border of the subscapularis tendon is seen between S and M.

The long head of the biceps brachii tendon originates from the posterosuperior labrum and supraglenoid tubercle. The biceps tendon plays an important role in stabilizing the humeral head during throwing.

Mechanisms of Labrum Injury

Various mechanisms have been postulated to cause glenoid labrum tears. Townley (23) thought that labral damage could occur from the same force that caused capsular avulsion or be secondary to repeated overriding of the humeral head once instability has developed. Bankart and Cantab (3) believed that anterior labral detachment most often originated from a fall backwards in which the humeral head was forced anteriorly, causing a shearing of the labrum. Other authors (16, 21) thought that a fall on the abducted externally rotated arm was the most common mechanism of anterior labral injury.

Pappas et al. (17) suggested that symptomatic labral tears without associated glenohumeral joint instability occur more frequently in heavily muscled and "tight jointed" individuals participating in strenuous activity. He described abduction, extension, and external rotation as the most common position of the shoulder at which anterior labral injury occurred, and a force along the longitudinal axis of the humerus with the shoulder in forward flexion to be the usual cause of posterior labral tears. He further theorized that inherent muscle strength in these patients served to prevent dislocation.

Andrews and Carson (1) have implicated the long head of the biceps tendon in the etiology of labral tears. They have suggested that an avulsion of the antero-superior labrum can occur from traction from the biceps tendon transmitted to the labrum, especially in the forceful throwing motion.

Diagnosis of Injury

A torn glenoid labrum usually causes symptoms when the shoulder goes to an extreme limit of motion. The most common syndrome is an anterior labrum tear resulting in catching or popping when the arm is overhead and goes into maximum external rotation, such as in pitching a baseball. If the shoulder subluxates in this position, the athlete may feel a sharp "paralyzing" pain and have a sensation that the arm goes "dead." The direction of subluxation or dislocation of the humeral head determines the location of tearing of the labrum: anterior instability results in a tear of the anterior labrum, inferior subluxation or dislocation tears the inferior labrum, and posterior instability tears the posterior labrum.

When a shoulder has a torn glenoid labrum, one should assume this was caused by glenohumeral instability until proven otherwise. Anatomically, the humeral head is much larger than the glenoid cavity and some subluxation may occur physiologically at extremes of motion. A baseball pitcher usually has more external rotation in abduction of the pitching arm than of the opposite shoulder. A loose-jointed individual also has a wide range of motion, and may even have physiological subluxation. In a study by Rowe and Zarins (22) of patients who had the dead arm syndrome, the diagnosis of subluxation was neither made by the patient nor the referring physician in half the cases that eventually were found to have the typical pathological findings of shoulder instability.

The association of labral injury and glenohumeral instability is analogous to the association of meniscal tears and knee instability. A torn anterior cruciate ligament results in recurrent anterior tibial subluxation that can tear the posterior third of a meniscus. The torn meniscus now can cause symptoms independent of the instability, and removing the torn meniscus can improve these symptoms without improving the subluxation. In fact, the knee can be more unstable after the meniscus is gone. Likewise, a shoulder can subluxate and this will tear the labrum. The shoulder can now click and pop with motion because of the interposing torn labrum. Removing the torn labrum can improve these symptoms, but potentially the shoulder will still be unstable.

Labral pathology associated with obvious glenohumeral instability often can be diagnosed by history and physical examination (18, 22). In these patients, a clear history of a dead arm can be correlated with a positive apprehension sign to reliably confirm the diagnosis.

However, not all patients with shoulder subluxation or symptomatic labral tears present with such clear-cut histories or definitive physical findings. Therefore, when the diagnosis is suspected but not confirmed by examination, additional studies are needed to confirm this diagnosis.

Protzman (18) has stated that most cases of shoulder subluxation could be diagnosed by appropriate plain radiographs. Rokous et al. (20) described the modified axillary or "West Point view" of the glenoid as a more reliable method of detecting anterior glenoid rim pathology. However, plain radiographs are only of value in cases that have bony pathology, and they will not reveal soft tissue pathology alone. Neer and Foster (16) described the use of stress radiographs to diagnose subtle glenohumeral instability. Other radiographic techniques that may be useful include arthrography, arthrotomography and computed tomography (CT) scanning.

Mizuno and Hiorhata (14) described the use of arthrography in combination with specialized radiographic projections of the shoulder to demonstrate labral pathology. They reported 35 cases in which labral lesions were demonstrated arthrographically and confirmed at the time of surgery. Braunstein and O'Connor (5) and Mink et al. (13) utilized double-contrast arthrography to demonstrate labral pathology. In 16 cases in which labral tears were demonstrated, 9 had surgery, at which time all were confirmed to have significant pathology. El-Khoury et al. (9) and McGlynn et al. (12) reported on the usefulness of arthrotomography of the glenoid labrum to demonstrate labral pathology (Figure 4–2). Pappas et al. (17) also utilized the technique of axillary arthrotomography as described by El-Khoury to demonstrate successfully labral pathology in patients in whom no associated glenohumeral instability was present.

Danzig et al. (7) have also reported on the use of CT scanning in combination with arthrographic techniques of the shoulder to demonstrate labral pathology. Nuclear magnetic resonance techniques may also play a future role in the diagnosis of labral pathology.

Our approach is to perform the appropriate history, physical examination, and plain radiographic evaluation in all patients with shoulder symptoms. If the shoulder clearly has instability, we will treat the instability rather than pursue further investigation of the labrum. If the direction of instability is uncertain, we usually perform arthroscopy to determine the probable direction of humeral head subluxation. If the patient has symptoms referable to the glenohumeral joint but no apparent subluxation, we usually proceed with arthroscopy as the next step. On occasion, we also utilize axillary arthrotomography to provide more information on the bony glenoid rim and the labrum.

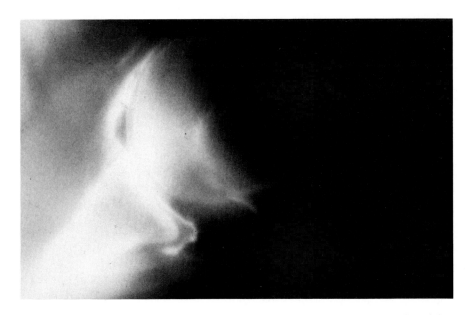

Figure 4–2 Axillary arthrotomogram showing a Bankart lesion at the anterior edge of the glenoid.

Arthroscopic Evaluation

Arthroscopy has several advantages over other techniques in diagnosing tears of the glenoid labrum. Direct visualization of the labrum allows a high degree of accuracy in diagnosis. The exact configuration and location of the labral tear can be determined. The condition of the articular surfaces and synovium can also be evaluated. Finally, definitive treatment of certain tears can be accomplished using arthroscopic surgical techniques at the same time as the arthroscopic examination (Figure 4–3). Arthroscopy has the disadvantages of being an invasive procedure and requiring general anesthesia.

Arthroscopic Anatomy

Shoulder arthroscopy can be performed in the operating room on an outpatient basis. Details of the technique of shoulder arthroscopy are described in the literature (2, 6, 11). General anesthesia with endotracheal intubation is usually used. The patient is positioned in the lateral decubitus position, and skin traction is used to apply 10 pounds of traction via a weight-and-pulley system.

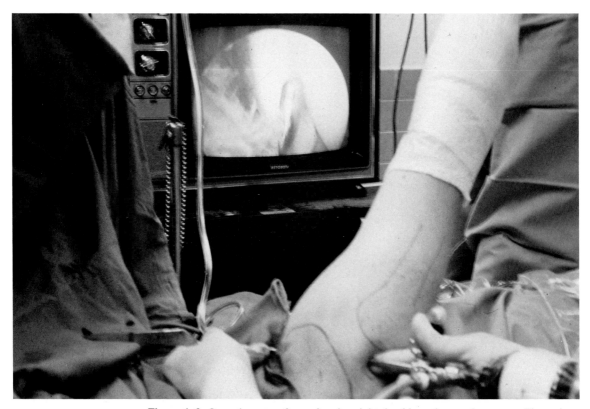

Figure 4–3 Operating setup for performing right shoulder arthroscopic surgery. The patient is in the lateral decubitus position with the right side up. The right arm is suspended in skin traction. The arthroscope has been introduced through a posterior portal and a probe has been inserted through an anterior portal. The suction and irrigation are connected to the arthroscope sheath. The procedure is being monitored on the video screen.

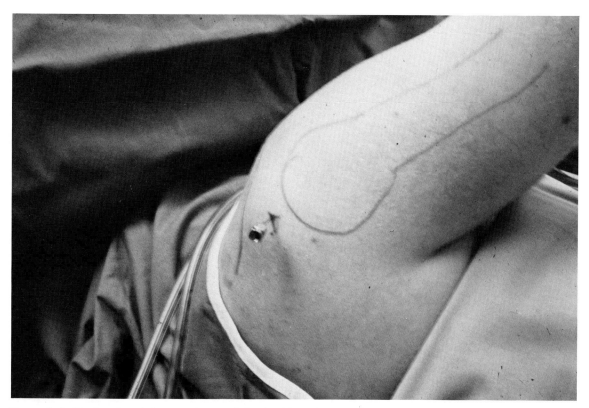

Figure 4–4 The location of the posterior portal for shoulder arthroscopy is 2 cm distal to the acromial angle at the posterior border of the deltoid muscle. The spinal needle has been introduced and is aimed toward the coracoid process anteriorly.

The posterior portal is located 2 cm distal to the acromial angle at a "soft spot" near the posterior edge of the deltoid muscle (Figure 4–4). The joint is first distended with saline introduced through a spinal needle. A 4- or 5-mm, 30-degree fore-oblique arthroscope is used for visualization. A television camera can be attached to the arthroscope to allow viewing on a video monitor.

The entire glenoid labrum can usually be well visualized using the standard posterior arthroscopy portal (Figure 4–5). The biceps tendon appears to blend with the posterosuperior labrum at the origin of the tendon from the supraglenoid tubercle (Figure 4–5, A). The labrum is usually largest and best defined anteriorly. The anterior labrum normally appears to be flat and to have a firm attachment that "blends" with the articular cartilage of the glenoid. There are three distinct thickenings of the anterior capsule, known as glenohumeral ligaments (Figure 4–1). The superior glenohumeral ligament is indistinct when viewed through the arthroscope in many shoulders. The middle glenohumeral ligament attaches to the anterior glenoid rim just distal to the upper border of the subscapularis tendon; there is variation in its normal anatomy. The inferior glenohumeral ligament attaches to the anteroinferior glenoid rim where it blends with the anterior labrum, from which it is frequently indistinguishable.

Inferiorly and posteriorly, the labrum is less well defined, yet is usually still a distinct structure (Figure 4–5, B). Minor irregularities of the posterior labrum are common.

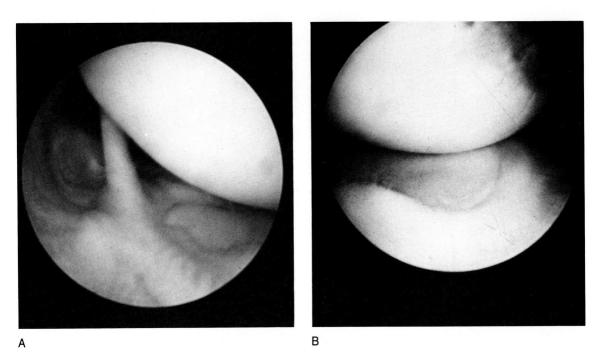

A   B

Figure 4–5 **A** Arthroscopic view, right shoulder seen from the posterior portal. The humeral head is on the upper right and the supraspinatus tendon is on the left. The biceps tendon spans the joint, taking origin from the supra glenoid tubercle. **B** Inferior and posterior glenoid labrum.

Tears

A description of a tear in the glenoid labrum should include the following information: 1) the *location* of the lesion (e.g., posterior, anterosuperior, anteroinferior, etc.); 2) the *configuration* or direction of the tear (e.g., flap tear, vertical longitudinal tear); and 3) associated capsular disruption, glenoid fracture, or other indicator of glenohumeral instability.

Most labrum tears occur in the anterosuperior quadrant or in the anterior third of the glenoid (1, 17). Less frequently, the inferior or posterior labrum can be disrupted.

The most common type of tear is a vertical longitudinal or circumferential tear (Figure 4–6). This is analogous to a bucket-handle tear of a knee meniscus. A flap tear is also frequently seen; this type of tear is a combination of a radial or oblique tear and a circumferential tear (Figure 4–7). Also seen is a labrum that has multiple interconnecting tears, making recognition of a predominant pattern difficult (Figure 4–8).

Disruption of the capsule and the attached labrum from the bony glenoid (Bankart lesion) suggests prior dislocation or subluxation of the humeral head (Figure 4–9). The location of the glenoid lesion correlates with the direction of excess excursion of the humeral head. For example, a circumferential tear of the inferior labrum suggests inferior glenohumeral subluxation (Figure 4–10). A fracture of the anterior glenoid rim plus a Hill-Sachs lesion of the humeral head are strong evidence of prior anterior dislocation.

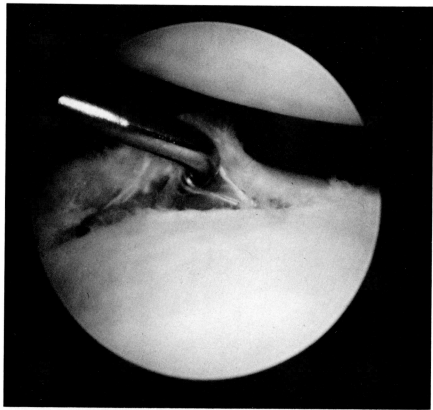

Figure 4–6 Arthroscopic view, right shoulder. The probe is lifting up the labrum, showing a vertical longitudinal (circumferential) tear in the anterior labrum.

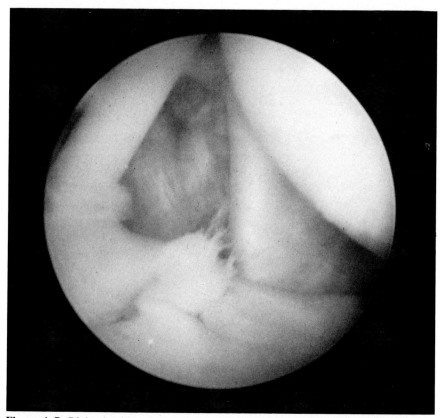

Figure 4–7 Right shoulder, flap tear of the anterosuperior portion of the labrum between the biceps tendon (left) and subscapularis tendon and rounded humeral head (right).

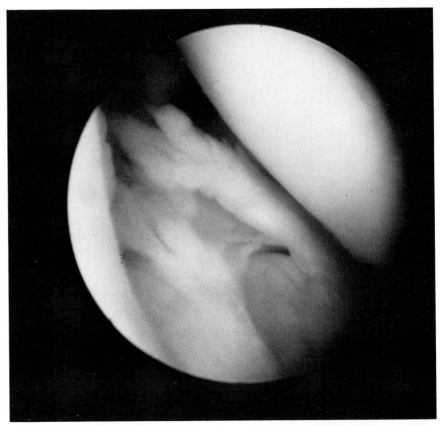

Figure 4–8 Complex tear, anterior labrum in a patient with recurrent posterior shoulder dislocations. This same shoulder had a circumferential tear of the posterior labrum.

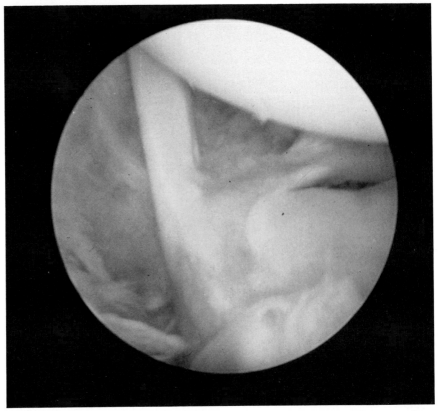

Figure 4–9 Bankart lesion, right shoulder. The anterior labrum and capsule have been avulsed from the anterior glenoid at the 3 o'clock position of this photograph.

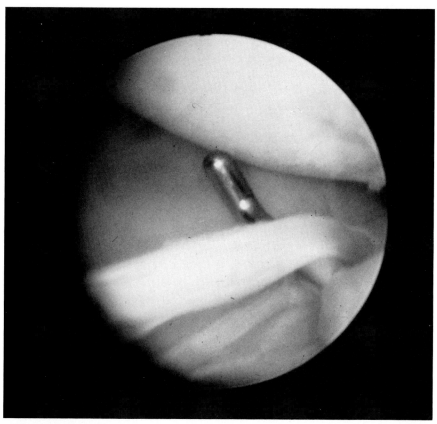

Figure 4–10 Right shoulder. The inferior labrum is torn in a circumferential manner, suggesting inferior glenohumeral subluxation. The probe is lifting the torn labrum, which has remained attached at both ends.

Vertical longitudinal (circumferential) tears are most often associated with recognizable shoulder subluxation. These are usually located anteriorly, anteroinferiorly, or posteriorly, depending on the type of instability. Flap tears are most commonly seen in shoulders of throwing athletes in which there is no apparent subluxation. Flap tears are most common in the anterosuperior quadrant. Traction of the biceps tendon on the labrum is implicated as a cause of injury (1).

Treatment

Nonoperative treatment of a torn labrum consists of symptomatic measures and avoidance of extremes of shoulder motion, especially abduction-external rotation (as in pitching a baseball). If the shoulder also subluxates, rotator cuff strengthening exercises can be of benefit.

Shoulder arthrotomy for excision of a torn labrum has been reported by Pappas et al. (17) to be successful in improving symptoms in shoulders that have functional (but not anatomical) instability due to a torn labrum. More recently, Andrews and Carson (1) have shown that arthroscopic resection of a torn labrum can improve shoulder symptoms in throwing athletes.

We utilize arthroscopic surgical methods for simple excision of a torn labrum and open arthrotomy in instances in which a Bankart procedure or capsulorrhaphy is to be done also. The technique of arthroscopic resection of a torn anterior labrum consists of using a motorized meniscotome introduced through an anterosuperior portal while visualizing with an arthroscope from the posterior portal (1, 2, 6, 11). The anterosuperior portal is located above and lateral to the coracoid process. The light from the arthroscope transilluminating the anterior shoulder between these intra-articular landmarks is a useful guide to correct placement of the anterior portal (Figure 4–11). A spinal needle introduced into the joint can be used to confirm the correct location of the portal before the incision is made. The incision enters the joint distal to the biceps tendon but proximal to the superior border of the sub-scapularis tendon (Figure 4–12).

The motorized meniscotome, basket biopsy forceps, or other arthroscopic instruments can be used to resect loose or unstable pieces of glenoid labrum. In resecting the torn labrum, care should be taken to leave stabilizing structures such as the glenohumeral ligaments intact. If the shoulder clearly has instability as a preexisting problem, simple resection of a torn labrum usually will not correct the problem (Figure 4–13). Consideration should be given to also performing a procedure that will correct the instability. We prefer the Bankart procedure (21, 22) for anterior or anteroinferior instability if a Bankart lesion exists. In cases of instability in which no Bankart lesion is found, anterior capsulorrhaphy is performed.

Intra-articular staples are now available for reattaching a torn labrum and capsule to the glenoid using arthroscopic methods. This technique is still unproven

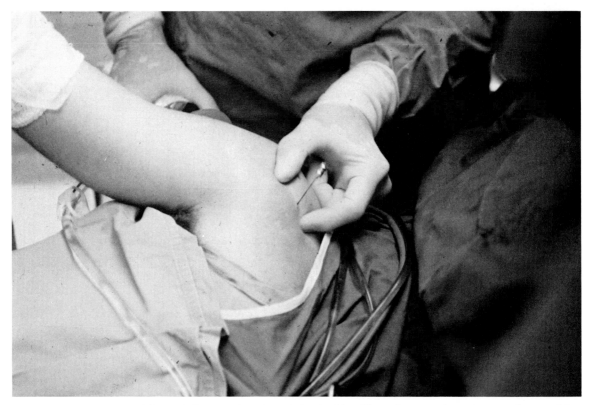

Figure 4–11 Anterior view, right shoulder. The arthroscope from the posterior portal is pushed against the skin anteriorly, transilluminating the skin. The light aids in correct placement of the anterior portal, which should be *lateral* to the coracoid process.

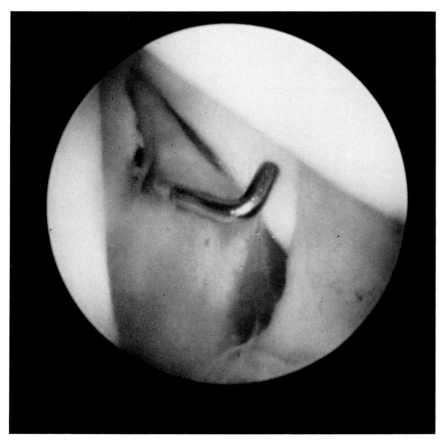

Figure 4–12 Intra-articular location of the anterior portal for arthroscopic surgery. The probe has been introduced between the biceps tendon (left) and superior border of subscapularis (right, at tip of probe). The humeral head is at the upper right.

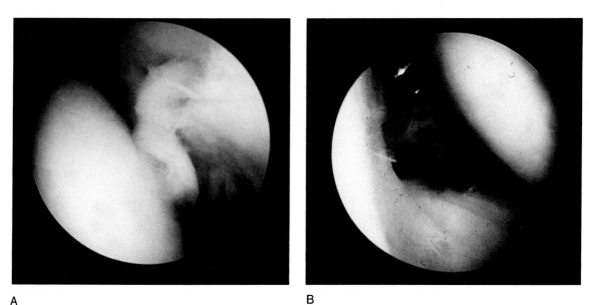

A   B

Figure 4–13 **A** Complex tear, anterior labrum, right shoulder in a professional hockey player. **B** Same shoulder following arthroscopic resection of the torn labrum. The patient continued to have symptoms although there was no recognizable subluxation. A Bankart procedure was performed. The patient has full range of motion and a stable shoulder at 2 years following surgery and is still playing professional hockey.

in effectiveness and carries significant potential risks because of the large protruding staple near the humeral head. We do not recommend this technique but prefer an open procedure, such as the Bankart technique, to correct anterior shoulder instability.

References

1. Andrews J, Carson W. The arthroscopic treatment of glenoid labrum tears in the throwing athlete. Orthop Trans 8:44, 1984
2. Andrews J, Carson W, Oretega K. Arthroscopy of the shoulder: technique and normal anatomy. Am J Sports Med 12:1–8, 1984
3. Bankart ASB, Cantab MC. Recurrent habitual dislocation of the shoulder joint. Br Med J 1132–1134, 1923(2)
4. Blazina ME, Satzman JS. Recurrent anterior subluxation of the shoulder in athletes— A distinct entity. J Bone Joint Surg [Am] 51:1037–1038, 1969
5. Braunstein EM, O'Connor G. Double-contrast arthrotomography of the shoulder. J Bone Joint Surg [Am] 64:192–195, 1982
6. Caspari RB. Shoulder arthroscopy: A review of the present state of the art. Contemp Orthop 4:523–530, 1982
7. Danzig L, Resnick D, Greenway G. Evaluation of unstable shoulders by computed tomography—A preliminary study. Am J Sports Med 10:138–142, 1982
8. DePalma AF. Surgery of the Shoulder, 2nd ed. JB Lippincott, Philadelphia, 1973
9. El-Khoury GY, Albright JP, Abu-Yousef MM, et al. Arthrotomography of the glenoid labrum. Radiol 131:333–337, 1979
10. Lombardo SJ. Arthroscopy of the shoulder. Clinics in Sports Medicine 2:309–318, 1983
11. Matthews LS, Vetter WL, Helfet DL. Arthroscopic surgery of the shoulder. Advances in Orthopaedic Surgery 7:203–210, 1984
12. McGlynn FJ, El-Khoury G, Albright JP. Arthrotomography of the glenoid labrum in shoulder instability. J Bone Joint Surg [Am] 64:506–518, 1982
13. Mink JH, Richardson A, Grant TT. Evaluation of glenoid labrum by double-contrast shoulder arthrography. AJR 133:883–887, 1979
14. Mizuno K, Hiorhata K. Diagnosis of recurrent traumatic anterior subluxation of the shoulder. Clin Orthop 179:160–167, 1983
15. Moseley HF, Overgaard B. The anterior capsular mechanism in recurrent anterior dislocation of the shoulder. J Bone Joint Surg [Br] 44:913–927, 1962
16. Neer CS II, Foster CR. Inferior capsular shift for involuntary inferior and multidirectional instability of the shoulder. J Bone Joint Surg [Am] 62:897–908, 1980.
17. Pappas AM, Goss TP, Kleinman PK. Symptomatic shoulder instability due to lesions of the glenoid labrum. Am J Sports Med 11:279–288, 1983
18. Protzman RR. Anterior instability of the shoulder. J Bone Joint Surg [Am] 62:909–918, 1980
19. Rockwood CA Jr. Subluxation of the shoulder. The classification, diagnosis and treatment. Orthop Trans 4:306, 1980
20. Rokous JR, Feagin JA, Abbott HG. Modified axillary roentgenogram. Clin Orthop 82:84–86, 1972
21. Rowe CR, Patel D, Southmayd WW. The Bankart procedure: A long term end-result study. J Bone Joint Surg [Am] 60:1–15, 1978
22. Rowe CR, Zarins B. Recurrent transient subluxation of the shoulder. J Bone Joint Surg [Am] 63:863–871, 1981
23. Townley CO. The capsular mechanism in recurrent dislocations of the shoulder. J Bone Joint Surg [Am] 32:370–380, 1950
24. Turkel SJ, Panio MW, Marshall JL et al. Stabilizing mechanisms preventing anterior dislocation of the glenohumeral joint. J Bone Joint Surg [Am] 63:1208–1217, 1981

Surgery for Recurrent Posterior Subluxation of the Shoulder

5

Richard J. Hawkins
Gary W. Misamore

Posterior instability of the shoulder is relatively uncommon. Acute traumatic posterior dislocation is rare and often may not be initially diagnosed, resulting in chronic or missed posterior dislocation. The large majority of patients with posterior instability of the shoulder, particularly in a young athletic population, have recurrent posterior subluxations rather than actual dislocations. It is the problem of recurrent posterior subluxation that is the topic of this discussion. This pathology is commoner than has been reported in the literature.

There are structural differences between the anterior and posterior aspects of the shoulder (7, 12). These anatomical differences account for the clinical differences between anterior and posterior shoulder instability. The posterior glenoid labrum is not as prominent or structurally supportive as the anterior labrum. The anterior labrum is reinforced by the glenohumeral ligaments, providing a definite degree of stability to the joint. Such reinforcing ligaments are absent posteriorly, although the anteroinferior glenohumeral ligament provides a degree of posterior stability through its global nature. The infraspinatus and teres minor are more muscular at the level of the glenohumeral joint and provide less support than the more tendinous subscapularis anteriorly. An understanding of these anatomical differences is important in understanding the clinical differences and the surgical treatment of posterior instability as compared to anterior instability.

Several developmental deformities, such as retroversion of the humeral head and glenoid, glenoid deficiency, and hyperlaxity of the capsule, may occasionally predispose to posterior instability of the shoulder (6, 8, 18, 24).

Previous classifications of recurrent shoulder instability have been confusing. Terms such as habitual, voluntary, involuntary, willful, intentional, unintentional, traumatic, and atraumatic have been used by various authors. The most important aspect to these classifications is the distinction of those patients with personality or psychiatric disorders. These habitual, willful subluxers can voluntarily sublux their shoulders but have little actual functional disturbance. Surgical treatment in these patients is fraught with failure. Treatment of their psychoemotional problems is the best management (23). Fortunately, in our experience, these psychiatrically disturbed patients with posterior instability are rare (13).

The large majority of patients with posterior instability are able to voluntarily subluxate their shoulders and have no psychiatric disorders. These patients should not be confused with the habitual, willful psychiatric subluxers. Most of the patients also have involuntary or unintentional subluxations of the shoulder during routine activities of daily living or during certain sporting activities in which the arm is placed in the flexed position. The involuntary subluxations may or may not be painful or functionally disabling for the patient. Most of these patients first develop unintentional or involuntary subluxation and eventually learn that with selective muscle action or by special positioning of the arm, posterior subluxation can be reproduced. This does not imply psychiatric disorders, and these patients should not be denied treatment simply because they have learned the mechanism necessary to reproduce their problem.

The final group of recurrent posterior subluxers consists of those who present with unintentional or involuntary subluxations and are incapable of demonstrating the instability. Diagnosis in these patients is extremely difficult. This is especially so now that we realize many normal patients have as much as 50% posterior translation of the humeral head in the glenoid, often more obvious under anesthesia. These patients are not often encountered since most have learned how to voluntarily subluxate the shoulder by the time they are seen by a physician.

Unlike patients with recurrent anterior dislocations, the majority of patients with recurrent posterior instability do not present with an initial episode of a traumatic dislocation requiring reduction (13). They often observe that following a specific strenuous activity or a traumatic injury to the shoulder, by certain movement of the arm, their shoulder "slips out of joint" and then easily reduces. In our experience, patients usually are accurate in identifying instability in their shoulders and generally are correct when they claim that the shoulder feels as though it slips out of joint. However, they often find it difficult to accurately distinguish direction. They may eventually learn to reproduce the instability by selective muscular contraction. The patient who can voluntarily sublux, by positioning the arm or by muscular contraction, almost always suffers from posterior instability, very rarely inferior, and almost never anterior. It is unusual for patients with posterior subluxations of the shoulder to complain of significant pain. It is also unusual for these patients to have such a functional disability that activities of daily living or work are significantly limited. However, it is not uncommon for patients with posterior instability to have interference with sports performance. In spite of this, many patients are able to throw, even though the shoulder subluxes during the overhead throwing-type of motion. This may only cause a minor abnormality with the overhead motion with very little discomfort. However, that difference from normal may produce a major performance change for high-caliber athletes.

Physical Examination

The most significant aspect of physical examination is the demonstration of posterior instability by the patient who subluxes the shoulder by selective muscle contraction or positioning of the arm. Many patients can sublux the shoulder posteriorly with the arm adducted at the side by contracting the internal rotator muscles. Other patients can readily reproduce the instability by placing the arm in the position that they have recognized as the most unstable for the shoulder. The position of the arm in which subluxation occurs is variable but usually involves forward elevation and internal rotation. Most commonly, posterior subluxation occurs when the arm is flexed between 30 and 100 degrees. With either more or less flexion, the shoulder spontaneously relocates. It is the relocation or reduction that is dramatically observed. The examiner should not be fooled by the occasional patient who puts the arm in the externally rotated and abducted position and yet can sublux the shoulder, not anteriorly as might be expected, but posteriorly. Diagnosis is very difficult in those patients with only involuntary, unintentional subluxation who are not able to voluntarily demonstrate posterior instability.

A positive "apprehension sign" is an important finding in recurrent anterior instability of the shoulder. In contrast, an apprehension sign is usually not reliable in recurrent posterior instability. Anterior instability cannot readily be demonstrated either actively by the patient or passively by the examiner. Beware of any additional component of inferior instability, which should alert the examiner to a diagnosis of multidirectional instability (20).

Radiographs

Plain radiographs are generally normal, but occasionally minor abnormalities can be identified that are suggestive of posterior subluxations (6). Avulsion fractures from the glenoid rim and impression defects in the humeral head, often seen in anterior instability, are unusual in patients with recurrent posterior subluxations. Radiographs in the lateral scapular view or the axillary view taken with the shoulder subluxed confirm the diagnosis. Arthrography is not diagnostic but may show an enlarged capsular pouch posteriorly. In doubtful cases arthroscopy may be useful to rule out anterior labral or glenoid rim defects or a Hill-Sachs lesion suggestive of anterior instability.

Treatment

Fortunately, most patients with posterior subluxation do not have sufficient pain or functional disability to justify surgical treatment. It is important to ensure that any pain or disability present is actually due to the instability and that it is truly a significant problem for the patient before attempting any surgical reconstruction. Many patients obtain relief of discomfort and lessening of the instability with rotator, especially external rotator, muscle strengthening. Those patients with voluntary subluxations due to psychiatric disorders should receive psychiatric treatment.

Surgical options include repair of posterior labral defects [reverse Bankart (1)], posterior staple capsulorraphy [reverse Dutoit (19, 28)], posterior capsular plication [reverse Putti-Platt, (22, 27)], transplantation of the long head of the biceps [modified Nicola (15, 21)], biceps tendon transfer combined with posterior soft tissue plication [Boyd-Sisk (14)], posterior bone block [reverse Eden-Hybbinette (9, 14)], glenoid osteotomy (3, 10, 22, 26), subscapularis transfer [McLaughlin (16, 17)], fascial slings [reverse Gallie (2, 11)], humeral osteotomy (2, 5), and inferior capsular shift (20). Reports of the results of the various surgical procedures for recurrent posterior instability have been varied. The complication and recurrence rates following some procedures have been relatively high. Rehabilitation following any of the surgical procedures is critical in achieving the return of good function to the operated shoulder and takes a long time.

Very few surgeons have had a large experience with surgery for recurrent posterior subluxation. Most reports of surgical reconstruction for this particular problem have dealt with very limited numbers of patients. Few statistically significant reports have been published, and no comparative studies of various treatment modalities can be found in the literature. Most reports of good results following surgical reconstruction for posterior subluxations have been based on the subjective impressions or personal opinions of the authors rather than on objective data.

It is essential that individuals treating instability about the shoulder appreciate the potential complexity of this disorder. Although some papers on repairs for posterior instability report good results, our recent experience has made us approach posterior instability with a guarded prognosis from a surgical point of view (13). A potential cause for failure in any shoulder procedure for instability is missing a diagnosis of direction or of more than one direction, i.e., multidirectional instability.

Combined posterior bone block and soft tissue plication is utilized by some to stabilize recurrent posterior instability. In the presence of glenoid deficiency, this procedure may be indicated. We have had little personal experience with posterior bone block other than in the above circumstances.

Glenoid osteotomy is a relatively popular procedure for this clinical entity. To condemn or promote this procedure would be unfair. One should be aware, however, that in the infrequent case of excessive retroversion of the glenoid, the osteotomy may be applicable. Our experience with glenoid osteotomies has been somewhat disappointing in that we have had several patients who have sustained intraoperative fractures of the glenoid with resultant joint incongruity and subsequent osteoarthritis of the glenohumeral joint. In fairness to the procedure, other authors have reported favorable results and are happy with the operation (3, 10, 22, 26). If this operation is to be employed, particular care must be taken to visualize the joint, keeping the osteotomy well away from the joint and taking it across to the opposite cortex.

Currently, our preference for surgical treatment of posterior instability consists of two approaches. At the time of surgery, the posterior tissues, particularly the inferior pouch, are assessed for substance, and a decision is made as to whether an inferior capsular shift, as described by Neer (20), will be sufficient or an additional procedure may be required. This procedure is combined with infraspinatus overlap. If the inferior capsule and pouch are of poor quality, the procedure is still performed with the appropriate infraspinatus overlap. However, a biceps tendon transfer, as popularized by Boyd and Sisk (4), is added. This procedure consists of transposing the biceps tendon, having detached it from the superior glenoid labrum, and passing it subperiosteally along the lateral aspect of the humeral head. Care must be taken to avoid injuring the axillary nerve. Concomitant to this transfer is the imbrication of the infraspinatus and teres minor tendons. The inferior capsular shift portion of the operation is designed to eliminate the redundant inferior capsular pouch. The free biceps tendon is then sutured to the repaired external rotators, theoretically providing a dynamic component to an essentially static repair. The results are fairly encouraging.

Unlike many shoulder procedures for which early motion is encouraged, with these operations we recommend rigid immobilization with a modified spica or prefabricated orthosis. The position employed is with the arm at the side in 20–30 degrees of external rotation. After spica removal the rehabilitation program works on rotational strengthening with a limited range of motion. Stretching to regain motion is delayed for 2–3 months.

The higher rates of recurrence and complications with surgical reconstruction for recurrent posterior subluxations than for anterior dislocations may be due to several factors. First, the relative infrequency of posterior instability requiring surgical reconstruction does not allow for the average surgeon to gain a great deal of experience with the problem. Second, the posterior soft tissues are less substantial than the anterior structures, making posterior reconstruction more technically demanding since a secure soft tissue repair is difficult to achieve. An additional problem may be the failure to recognize and appropriately treat multidirectional instability. Careful preoperative patient selection, careful adherence to appropriate surgical technique, and vigorous postoperative rehabilitation will maximize success.

Surgical reconstriction for recurrent posterior subluxation is a challenging problem. Fortunately, most patients with this problem do not require surgical intervention. Patients should be managed conservatively unless truly significant pain or functional disability exists. Recurrent posterior subluxation presents a great dilemma in athletic patients. Whether or not surgical intervention is beneficial or indicated in this situation remains an unanswered question. Our review of athletic performance following surgery for posterior instability has been disappointing overall. The soundness of undertaking a surgical reconstruction that has unproven results in an attempt to improve athletic performance is open to question. Our current approach to this situation emphasizes conservative treatment. Our attitude toward operative procedures for reconstruction of recurrent posterior subluxation remains guarded.

References

1. Bankart ASB. The pathology and treatment of recurrent dislocation of the shoulder joint. Br J Surg 26:23, 1938
2. Bateman JE. The Shoulder and Neck. WB Saunders, Philadelphia, 1978
3. Bestasrd EA. Genoplasty: A simple reliable method of correcting recurrent posterior dislocation of the shoulder. Orthop Rev 5:29, 1976
4. Boyd HB, Sisk TD. Recurrent posterior dislocation of the shoulder. J Bone Joint Surg [Am] 54:779, 1972
5. Chaudhier GR, Sengupta A, Saha AK. Rotation osteotomy of the shaft of the humerus for recurrent dislocation of the shoulder: Anterior and posterior. Acta Orthop Scand 45:193, 1974
6. Connolly J. X-ray defects in recurrent shoulder dislocations. J Bone Joint Surg [Am] 51:1235, 1969
7. DePalma AF. Surgery of the Shoulder. JB Lippincott, Philadelphia, 1983
8. Dogan JA. Posterior dislocation of the shoulder. Am J Surg 89:890, 1955
9. Eden R. Zur Operation der habitueller schulter Luxation unter Mitteilung zeines Verfahrens bei Agriss an innerer Pfamenrande. Deutsche Zeitschrift für Chirurgie 144:299, 1918
10. Edmonson AS, Crenshaw AH. Campbell's Operative Orthopedics, 6th ed. CV Mosby, St. Louis, 1980
11. Gallie WE, Lemesurier AB. Recurring dislocation of the shoulder. J Bone Joint Surg [Br] 30:9, 1948
12. Grant JCB. Grant's Atlas of Anatomy, 6th ed. Williams & Wilkins, Baltimore, 1972
13. Hawkins RJ, Koppert GJ. Recurrent posterior instability (subluxation) of the shoulder. J Bone Joint Surg 66:169, 1984
14. Hybbinette S. De la transplantation d'un fragment osseux pour remédier aux luxations récidivantes de l'épaule; Constatations et résultats opératoires. Acta Chir Scand 71:411, 1932

15. May H. Nicola operation for posterior subacromial dislocation of the humerus. J Bone Joint Surg 25:78, 1943

16. McLaughlin HL. Posterior dislocation of the shoulder. J Bone Joint Surg [Am] 34:584, 1952

17. McLaughlin HL. Posterior dislocation of the shoulder. J Bone Joint Surg [Am] 44:1477, 1962

18. Mollerud A. A case of bilateral habitual luxation in the posterior part of the shoulder joint. Acta Chir Scand 94:181, 1946

19. Neer CS. Reconstructive surgery and rehabilitation of the shoulder. In: Kelly WN et al. Textbook of Rheumatology, pp 1944–1959. WB Saunders, Philadelphia, 1981

20. Neer CS, Foster CR. Inferior capsular shift for involuntary inferior and multidirectional instability of the shoulder. A preliminary report. J Bone Joint Surg [Am] 63:416, 1981

21. Nicola T. Recurrent dislocation of the shoulder: Its treatment by transplantation of the long head of the biceps. Am J Surg 6:815, 1929

22. Rockwood CA, Green DP. Fractures and Dislocations. JB Lippincott, Philadelphia, 1972

23. Rowe CR, Pierce DS, Clark JG. Voluntary dislocation of the shoulder. A preliminary report on a clinical, electromyographic and psychiatric study of twenty-six patients. J Bone Joint Surg [Am] 55:445, 1973

24. Samilson RL, Miller E. Posterior dislocations of the shoulder. Clin Orthop 32:69, 1964

25. Samilson RL, Prieto V. Posterior dislocation of the shoulder in athletes. Clinics in Sports Medicine 2:369, 1983

26. Scott DJ. Treatment of recurrent posterior dislocations of the shoulder by glenoplasty. J Bone Joint Surg [Am] 49:471, 1967

27. Severin E. Anterior and posterior recurrent dislocations of the shoulder: The Putti-Platt operation. Acta Orthop Scand 23:14, 1953

28. Tibone JE, Prieto C, Jobe FW. Staple capsulorrhaphy for recurrent posterior shoulder dislocations. Am J Sports Med 9:135, 1981

Decompression of the Coracoacromial Arch

6

Douglas W. Jackson
Ben K. Graf

Chronic or recurrent subacromial shoulder pain is a common complaint in athletes of all ages. Impingement under the coracoacromial arch may be the basis for a specific symptom complex. Since impingement generally occurs between 60 and 120 degrees of shoulder elevation (12), it is not surprising that the impingement syndrome is frequently seen in the throwing athlete and in those involved in repetitive overhead activities. This latter group includes those participating in tennis, racquetball, handball, volleyball, gymnastics, and swimming (6). While most individuals with impingement will respond to conservative measures, some will require surgical intervention to enable them to return to their sport.

Surgical Anatomy

The shoulder is a multiaxial ball-and-socket joint with mobility in many planes but has a propensity for instability. The radius of curvature of the glenoid is approximately one-half that of the humeral head, resulting in a small area of bony contact. Even when the labrum is considered in the calculations, the diameter of the "socket" is less than two-thirds that of the humeral head (21). Therefore, capsular restraints and balanced muscular forces are essential to normal function of the shoulder. The prime movers of the shoulder, unless force coupled with the depressors of the rotator cuff (7), tend to compress the humeral head against the acromion and coracoacromial ligament. The long head of the biceps tendon may also act as a humeral head depressor. Thus, the rotator cuff and biceps tendon act as both

51

mechanical spacers and dynamic barriers to superior migration of the humeral head and concomitant impingement.

The roof of the shoulder joint is formed by a bony and fibrous arch—the acromion, coracoid process, coracoacromial ligament, and the undersurface of the acromioclavicular (AC) joint. The coracoacromial ligament is triangular in shape, originating from the broad lateral surface of the coracoid and inserting on a small area of the undersurface of the acromion. Its central fibers may be attenuated, leaving well-defined anterior and posterior bands (24). The humeral head, with the rotator cuff inserting on its prominent greater tuberosity, lies below the arch. In between these unyielding structures are the rotator cuff, the long head of the biceps tendon, and the subacromial bursa. The bursa sits like a cap on top of the rotator cuff, to which it is firmly attached. The largest bursa in the body, it sends an extension under the coracoid process. With abduction of the arm, its superior surface rolls across the fixed inferior surface. In this way it allows smooth, gliding motion between the greater tuberosity and rotator cuff, and the overlying deltoid and coracoacromial arch. The biceps tendon lies in a groove between the greater and lesser tuberosities and originates from superior lip of the glenoid labrum. With motion of the shoulder, the biceps remains fixed as the humerus moves around it. It is surrounded by a synovial extension of the glenohumeral joint to accommodate such motion. Since the bicipital groove is of variable depth and configuration, the transverse humeral ligament, which forms the roof of the groove, is an important restraint to bicipital tendon dislocation.

Pathophysiology

The impingement syndrome may develop when the available space is decreased or when the contents are increased in size. Repetitive microtrauma may result in inflammation, partial tearing, and thickening of the rotator cuff. The subacromial bursae may also be irritated, with thickening of their walls, accumulation of fluid, and adhesion formation. Synovitis and effusion can have many causes; both are space-occupying processes. Finally, calcium deposits may tip the balance from normal function to impingement.

Neer (14) has demonstrated excrescences and spurs involving the undersurface of the acromion in patients with impingement. Osteophytes on the undersurface of the AC joint may also be a causative factor.

Based on his clinical experience and a dissection of 100 cadavers, Neer described a critical area for impingement. He reported that the region of tendonitis and rupture is usually centered in the supraspinatus tendon, with variable extension to include the anterior portion of the infraspinatus and the long head of the biceps tendon (14). The area of most frequent involvement corresponds to the hypovascular area of the supraspinatus demonstrated by Rathbun and McNab (23). By diminishing the tendon's ability to repair itself, limited vascularity may play a role in the impingement syndrome.

With the arm in neutral rotation, the supraspinatus, anterior portion of the infraspinatus, and biceps all lie anterior to the coracoacromial arch. With internal rotation these structures come to lie even more anterior, and with external rotation the supraspinatus is just lateral to the acromion. Elevation of the arm causes the critical area to pass under anterior acromion and other components of the arch. According to Kessel and Watson (12), this process begins at approximately 60 degrees and is completed by 120 degrees, thus defining the impingement zone.

Clinical Stages

Three stages of impingement have been described (5, 15). Stage I is the stage of edema and hemorrhage. This reversible process generally occurs in individuals less than 25 years old but can occur at any age. Patients complain of an ache, usually felt anteriorly, which occurs after throwing or overhead activities.

Stage II is characterized by fibrosis and tendonitis and typically is seen in 25- to 40-year-olds. It is thought to result from repeated insults to the cuff and often causes pain with activity and also at night. Limitation of activity may not result in complete pain relief. Bicipital tendonitis is more common in this stage.

Stage III seldom occurs before age 40. Chronic impingement abrades the critical area, generating full- or partial-thickness cuff tears. Again, involvement of the biceps is common, but Neer (15) feels that the ratio of supraspinatus to biceps ruptures is 7:1. Signs of a rotator cuff tear such as weakness or atrophy of rotator cuff muscles may be present. Roentgenograms are frequently positive, with sclerosis and osteophyte formation at the anterior acromion, AC joint degenerative changes, cystic changes in the greater tuberosity, or superior migration of the humeral head.

Physical Exam

Since the general examination of the shoulder has been reviewed in Chapter 1, only those tests specific for the impingement syndrome will be described here.

A painful arc from 60 to 120 degrees of abduction is characteristic of a disorder of the coracoacromial arch. Limitation of motion is also significant since a small percentage of patients with impingement may develop a frozen shoulder. Tenderness over the greater tuberosity and along the course of the coracoacromial ligament is generally present. More often a finding in stage II or III, soft tissue crepitus may be felt and heard as the shoulder is internally and externally rotated with the arm flexed or abducted 90 degrees. This may represent scarring of the subacromial bursae in the early stages or actual bony impingement later on. Tenderness over the bicipital groove should be searched for as well as biceps tendon rupture.

Several provocative tests for impingement have been described. Forced elevation of the shoulder, with the scapula stabilized by the examiner's free hand, causes pain in all stages of impingement (15) (Figure 6–1, A). With the arm held in 90 degrees of flexion, forced internal rotation is also an effective method for reproducing the patient's pain (5) (Figure 6–1, B). Finally, resisted abduction with the arm abducted 90 degrees, horizontally flexed 30 degrees, and maximally internally rotated isolates the supraspinatus and frequently results in impingement pain (10) (Figure 6–1, C).

Injection of lidocaine into the subacromial bursae is a useful adjunct to the above tests. After the injection the pain with each of these maneuvers should be markedly reduced. The anesthetic is also useful in evaluating the function of the rotator cuff. The weakness secondary to pain commonly seen in those patients with impingement but without rotator cuff tears is generally alleviated by injection, whereas the true weakness associated with large cuff tears is unaffected.

Biceps tendonitis usually does not occur as a separate entity (18), but it is a frequent participant in the impingement syndrome. Tenderness over the biceps, especially just below the transverse humeral ligament, is essential to the diagnosis. The biceps resistance test is usually positive and is performed by resisting flexion

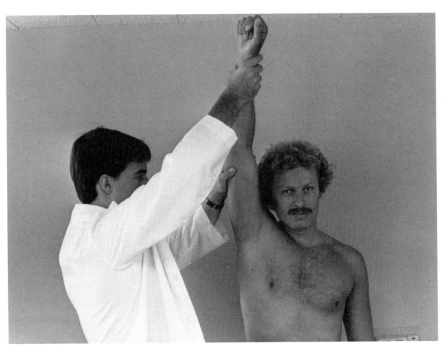

A

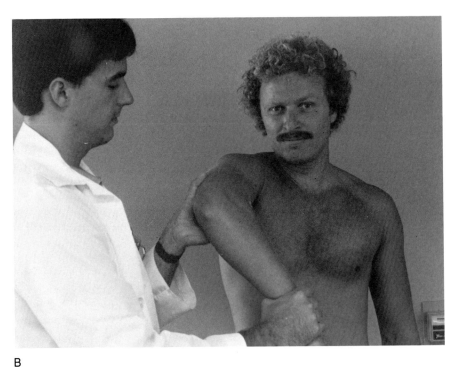

B

Figure 6–1

of the arm with the forearm supinated and the elbow extended (Figure 6–2). Biceps tendonitis is largely unaffected by injections of local anesthetic into the subacromial bursae since the biceps tendon is surrounded by a sheath that is an extension of the synovial lining of the glenohumeral joint, not the subacromial bursae.

A painful arc from 120 degrees of abduction to full abduction is more indicative of AC problems than the impingement syndrome. Forced adduction of the

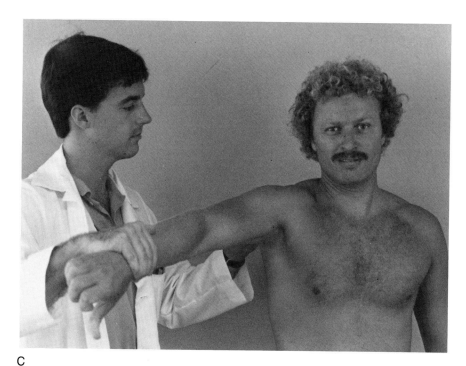

C

Figure 6–1 Impingement tests. **A** Forced elevation of the arm. **B** Flexion and forced internal rotation. **C** Resisted abduction in 30 degrees flexion, full internal rotation, and 90 degrees abduction.

arm across the chest is also effective in producing pain in those patients with degenerative changes of the AC joint. To define appropriate treatment, it is essential to differentiate AC joint pain from impingement pain.

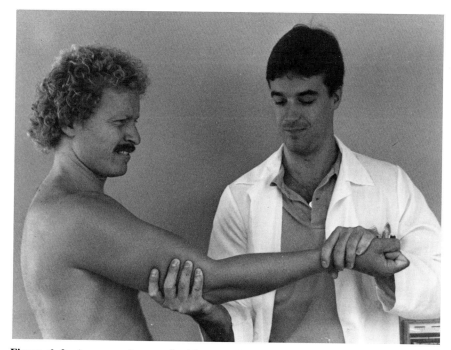

Figure 6–2 A provocative test for biceps tendonitis is resisted flexion of the supinated forearm.

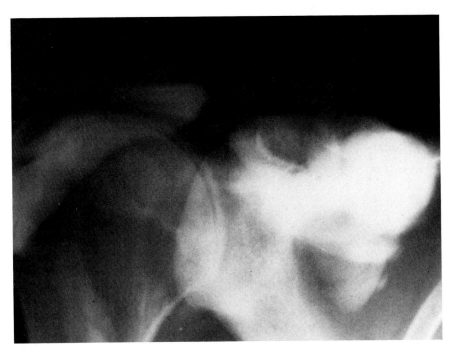

Figure 6–3 A normal bursagram/arthrogram.

Roentgenograms

In stage I or II, the roentgenograms are generally negative. In stage 3, however, anterior acromial spurs, spurring or cystic changes of the greater tuberosity, and degenerative changes of the AC joint may be present (2). With massive cuff tears eburnation of the acromion can occur as a result of superior migration of the humeral head. Arthrograms are helpful in patients with stage II or III disease who have failed conservative treatment, noted the sudden onset of rotator cuff weakness, or ruptured the long head of the biceps tendon. Weakness following a glenohumeral dislocation is also an indication for arthrography (16).

Subacromial bursography has its proponents (25). A normal subacromial bursa easily accepts 5–10 ml of contrast medium (Figure 6–3). Conversely, abnormal bursa either accept much less contrast or cannot be demonstrated at all. Conservative and operative treatment of presumed impingement has been found to be less successful in patients with normal bursagrams than in those with abnormal studies. Therefore, the diagnosis of impingement syndrome should be questioned in the presence of a normal bursagram.

Differential Diagnosis of Impingement Syndrome

Calcific Tendonitis

Acute, subacute, and chronic variants have been described. The acute form has the most dramatic presentation, with sudden onset of severe shoulder pain, exacerbated by any attempts at motion. The other variants have a more insidious onset. The calcium deposits are often seen on radiographs, although not on every view. During the acute, severely painful phase an attempt to percutaneously rupture the deposit can be made, although given the difficulty in localizing the lesion, this is a blind procedure. A corticosteroid injection is often effective, even when not associated with needling of the calcific area. Nonoperative management is usually successful and may require a few days of strong pain medication. Bedrest and sleeping in the semisitting position is often helpful during the acute phase. A minority of patients will require surgical incision and evacuation of their deposits. This is done through a small deltoid-splitting incision. Depalma (3) has reported good results in 96% of patients so treated.

Traumatic Bursitis

When the subdeltoid bursa is directly traumatized, as may occur when a football player is struck or lands on the apex of his shoulder, edema and hemorrhage of the bursa may occur. Appropriate initial treatment is rest and ice, followed in a few days by mobilization of the shoulder. Complete recovery in 2–3 weeks can be expected.

AC Joint Pathology

Acute and chronic AC joint problems are frequent causes of anterior shoulder pain. Local tenderness and discomfort with the appropriate provocative maneuvers are signs that should prompt further investigation.

Synovitis

Synovial thickening and joint effusion may themselves result in pain or may initiate an impingement phenomenon. Rheumatoid arthritis, other connective tissue diseases, gout, and pseudogout may be causes of unexplained, persistent, or recurrent synovitis. Early degenerative arthritis is difficult to diagnose. It can follow trauma such as a dislocation or have an insidious onset. A strenuous repetitive activity can place excessive demands on the glenohumeral joint and represent another etiology of pain, synovitis, and even effusion.

Glenohumeral Instability

Throwing athletes and swimmers, particularly backstrokers, are prone to instability problems. Differentiation of subtle presentations of this entity from impingement often proves to be difficult. Positive apprehension tests, a history of dislocations, feelings of subluxation, dead arm symptoms, and radiographic signs, such as a Hill-Sachs lesion or abnormal glenoid, are all suggestive of subluxation or dislocation. Occasionally, multiple examinations over an extended period of time are required to differentiate subtle instability from impingement. Arthroscopic or fluoroscopic examination, or examination under anesthesia may be necessary to prove the presence and direction of the instability.

Nonoperative Treatment

Most patients with impingement, especially those in stage I, can be successfully treated without surgery. A review of 480 patients seen in our clinic over a 5-year period revealed only 50 patients who failed to respond to conservative therapy. An effective nonoperative program is based on rest, anti-inflammatory medication, shoulder stretching and strengthening, and avoidance of reinjury.

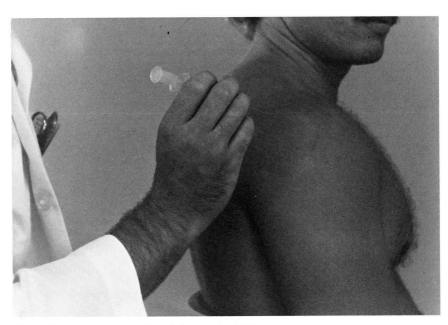

Figure 6–4 Posterior injection of the subacromial bursa.

Rest

Requisite to recovery in most instances is a period of avoidance of overhead or throwing activities. Cardiovascular fitness, and shoulder strength and flexibility need not be compromised. Swimmers may train with a kick board or change strokes for a few weeks. Pitchers will usually have to stop throwing for a time but can continue batting practice and are able to run or cycle for fitness. Similarly, laborers may be required to take time off from repetitive overhead activities at work. A common mistake is to return the patient too quickly to the aggravating activity.

Medications

During the rest period anti-inflammatory medication is often useful to speed the recovery. An injection into the subacromial bursa of a local anesthetic, combined with a steroid preparation, is a useful diagnostic and therapeutic maneuver (Figure 6–4). Such injections should not be repeated more than two or three times in any one year because of their potential effect on tendon strength. It may be, however, that short-acting preparations have less of a detrimental effect than long-acting ones (1). As an adjunct to injection, or a substitute for it, nonsteroidal anti-inflammatory medications have also proved useful. Such medications can be continued during the early rehabilitative phase to provide pain relief and prevent recurrence.

Rehabilitation

Shoulder stretching and strengthening programs should begin as soon as the acute inflammation has subsided. Specifics of such programs are covered in a later chapter.

Return to Function

Before returning the athlete to his preinjury activity level, it is important to check for proper body mechanics and form and to avoid errors in training and technique. Pitchers, for example, may place excessive loads on the shoulder by opening up too soon, i.e., letting the body turn towards the batter too early in the pitching motion. The natural response is to drop the elbow and short-arm the ball (19). Similarly, tennis players, swimmers, and others may have recurrence of impingement problems prevented by attention to proper technique.

It is also important that the return to the inciting activity be gradual. As an illustration, consider the program for pitchers outlined by Jobe (9). The player starts in the outfield, throwing the ball so that it reaches home plate after three or four bounces. He does not throw hard but uses his full throwing motion for about 15 minutes. The second day he may move a bit closer and throw slightly harder, letting the ball bounce only once or twice. The third day he throws with only one bounce and slowly works towards the mound. Once there he starts at half speed and gradually increases his velocity. The whole process may take 3 weeks for a rest period and an additional 3 weeks to work back into pitching. The return to other athletic endeavors should also be structured in a graduated manner.

Operative Management

Coracoacromial Ligament Resection

Indications Surgical treatment of the impingement syndrome should only be considered in those patients who have failed to respond to 6–12 months of conservative management and are unwilling or unable to sufficiently restrict their activities to alleviate their discomfort. Coracoacromial ligament resection as an isolated procedure has been proposed by several authors (4, 5, 8, 11, 22). It is most likely to be successful in patients with stage I impingement or those with stage II disease but no osseous abnormalities. It probably should not be considered alone for patients with rotator cuff tears since in a small series of 16 such patients, Penny and Welsh (20) found better results when cuff repair was combined with acromioplasty than when only repair and coracoacromial ligament resection was done. They also felt that bicipital tendonitis was successfully treated by coracoacromial ligament resection without any special attention to the biceps itself.

Technique Under local or general anesthesia the patient is placed in the semisitting position with the head turned away from the affected side and the arm and shoulder prepped and draped free. A short strap incision is made from the AC joint to a point just lateral to the coracoid. The deltopectoral fascia is incised, and the deltoid is bluntly divided in line with its fibers. The coracoacromial ligament is identified as a tough fibrous band with a sharp leading edge. It is generally quite broad at its coracoid origin and tapers to a smaller area of insertion on the acromion. Anterior and posterior bands may be present and both must be recognized. Prior to transection of the ligament, the shoulder is put through the impingement maneuvers; popping and grating are usually noted. The entire ligament is then resected along with the subacromial bursa if it is thickened. When the arm is once again rotated in 90 degrees of flexion or abduction, the popping should no longer be present. If the patient is awake, he usually can report that the impingement is gone. With traction applied to the arm, the undersurface of the acromion and AC joint can be palpated. Osteophytes, AC arthritis, or insufficient clearance between the humeral head and the acromion generally signal the need for a more aggressive decompres-

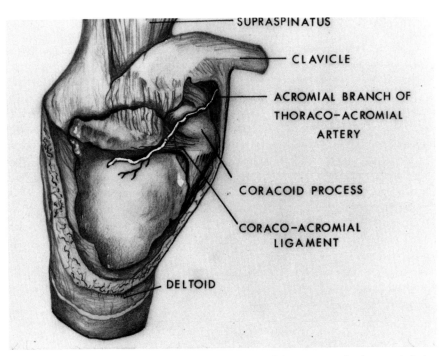

SUPRASPINATUS

CLAVICLE

ACROMIAL BRANCH OF
THORACO-ACROMIAL
ARTERY

CORACOID PROCESS

CORACO-ACROMIAL
LIGAMENT

DELTOID

Figure 6–5 The acromial branch of the thoracoacromial artery may be lacerated during coracoacromial ligament resection.

sion. The acromial branch of the thoracoacromial artery is frequently cut during this procedure (Figure 6–5). It can retract medially and be difficult to control without adequate exposure. This has been a problem on occasion for those who advocate dividing the ligament blindly or arthroscopically.

Postoperatively, the patient is kept in a sling for 3–5 days and then begun on passive range-of-motion exercises. If no deltoid has been detached from the acromion, active motion and strengthening can be initiated as pain allows; otherwise it is delayed 10–14 days to accommodate deltoid reattachment.

Anterior Acromioplasty

Indications Anterior acromioplasty is the procedure of choice in patients with stage III impingement who have failed conservative treatment. Some authors feel that it should always accompany ligament resection. Most agree that patients with osteophytes or those who at the time of surgery are felt to have insufficient clearance between the greater tuberosity or supraspinatus tendon and the acromion should undergo osseous decompression.

Individuals with impingement and AC joint arthritis represent a special situation. Resection of 1–2 cm of the distal clavicle in addition to decompression of the coracoacromial arch may be necessary to control symptoms (4, 13, 20). For this reason radiographic evaluation of the AC joint is recommended before any coracoacromial arch surgery. In those cases where the AC joint is enlarged but not degenerative, adequate decompression can be obtained by beveling the undersurface without resecting the joint (15). Finger palpation of the undersurface of the joint should assist in determining the extent of surgery.

Usually biceps tendonitis associated with impingement requires no treatment other than the indicated decompression. When the long head of the biceps is acutely ruptured, it should be tenodesed in its groove at the time of acromioplasty. Resection of the intra-articular portion is seldom necessary.

Technique (Neer) The technique of anterior acromioplasty described by Neer and Marberry (17) does not weaken the deltoid as many other acromionectomies have and is effective, since impingement is an anterior phenomenon. The patient is placed in the semisitting position with the arm draped free and the shoulder hanging over the edge of the table. An incision is begun at the posterior edge of the AC joint and extended anteriorly and inferiorly in line with the axillary skin crease to end just lateral to the coracoid. The deep fascia is incised, and the deltoid is split in line with its fibers 5 cm below the acromion. Further splitting will injure the axillary nerve. If indicated, the inferior capsule of the AC joint is incised, the deltoid and trapezius are elevated, and 1–2 cm of the distal clavicle is excised. The coracoacromial ligament is identified and resected. When required for exposure, deltoid fibers may be elevated from the anterior acromion, but such dissection should involve no more than 1 cm of deltoid attachment. A cuff of tissue should be left attached to the acromion to facilitate reattachment at the end of the procedure.

Soft tissues are dissected from the undersurface of the acromion and an oblique osteotomy is performed. An osteotome or oscillating saw is used to remove the anterior overhanging portion of the acromion. It may be helpful to have an assistant strike the osteotome, leaving the surgeon a free hand to palpate the acromion and gauge the thickness of the remaining superior portion. The cut surface is smoothed with a rongeur and all loose fragments of bone are removed. The shoulder is put through a range of motion to document that impingement is no longer present. The rotator cuff is carefully inspected and any tears are repaired. If acutely ruptured, the biceps tendon is tenodesed in its groove with multiple sutures.

When release has been necessary, the deltoid is reattached to the acromion with interrupted absorbable sutures. If the distal clavicle has been excised, the deltoid is sutured to the trapezius with mattress sutures. Prior to skin closure a small suction drain may be inserted.

Postoperatively, the patient may begin passive range-of-motion exercises as soon as the wound allows. Active forward flexion is prohibited for 10–14 days to allow the deltoid to reattach.

Arthroscopy

The use of the arthroscope is being defined in relation to the rotator cuff and has limited therapeutic value presently in impingement syndrome. Arthroscopic debridement of the undersurface of the rotator cuff has been advocated as a way to stimulate healing of partial-thickness tears. It may also be used for the removal of fibrous tissue resulting from abortive attempts at cuff repair. By introducing the arthroscope into the subacromial bursa it is possible to remove the bursal lining, resect the coracoacromial ligament, and even to remove a portion of the undersurface of the acromion. The latter is accomplished with a burr of the type used for abrasion chondroplasty. Whether or not these difficult procedures can be refined for widespread use remains to be seen.

Surgical Failure Following Decompression

The most common cause of a poor result following surgical decompression is an error in diagnosis. Subtle instability may be difficult to diagnose and may masquerade as impingement, with anterior shoulder pain, discomfort after throwing, and complaints of popping in the shoulder. Early glenohumeral degenerative arthritis may also present with symptoms similar to those seen with impingement. Underlying systemic connective tissue diseases can cause impingement, yet these patients may respond poorly to decompression.

Tenderness over the long head of the biceps tendon in a patient who has not responded to decompression should alert one to the possibility of biceps tendonitis. We have found that although bicipital tendonitis is usually relieved by decompression, this is not always the case. These patients may note dramatic improvement with biceps tenodesis.

Pain and popping in the anterior shoulder is occasionally caused by a subluxing biceps tendon. In nearly all cases a history of significant shoulder trauma can be obtained (24). Athletes rarely present with this problem.

An inadequate decompression is, in our experience, an uncommon reason for surgical failure, but can be caused by insufficient resection of bone or ligament. Most failures result from faulty diagnosis rather than inadequate surgery. There are, however, individuals who are asymptomatic for several years following surgery and then notice recurrence of their impingement symptoms. We have had success with repeat decompression in such cases.

References

1. Butler D, Noyes F, Grood E. Effects of intracollagenase injection of two corticosteroids on ligament/tendon properties. Paper presented at the 27th Annual Meeting of the Orthopaedic Research Society, Las Vegas, 1981
2. Cone R III, Resnick D, Danzig L. Shoulder impingement syndrome: Radiographic evaluation. Radiology 150:29–33, 1984
3. DePalma A. Surgery of the Shoulder, 3rd ed, p 277. JB Lippincott, Philadelphia, 1983
4. Ha'eri G, Wiley AM. Shoulder impingement syndrome: Results of operative release. Clin Orthop 168:128–132, 1982
5. Hawkins RJ, Kennedy JC. Impingement syndrome in athletes. Am J Sports Med 8:151–158, 1980
6. Hill JA. Epidemiologic perspective on shoulder injuries. Clinics in Sports Medicine 2:241–246, 1983
7. Inman V, Saunders JB, Abbott LC. Observations on the function of the shoulder joint. J Bone Joint Surg 26:1–30, 1944
8. Jackson DW. Chronic rotator cuff impingement in the throwing athlete. Am J Sports Med 4:231–240, 1976
9. Jobe FW. Thrower problems. Sports Med 7:139–144, 1979
10. Jobe FW, Jobe CM. Painful athletic injuries of the shoulder. Clin Orthop 173:117–124, 1983
11. Johansson JE, Barrington TW. Coracoacromial ligament division. Am J Sports Med 12:138–141, 1984
12. Kessel L, Watson M. The painful arc syndrome. J Bone Joint Surg [Br] 59:166–172, 1977
13. Misamore GW, Hawkins RJ. Shoulder impingement syndrome: When to suspect, what to do. Journal of Musculoskeletal Medicine 55–63, July, 1984
14. Neer CS II. Anterior acromioplasty for the chronic impingement syndrome in the shoulder: A preliminary report. J Bone Joint Surg. [Am] 54:41–50, 1972
15. Neer CS II. Impingement lesions. Clinical Orthop 173:70–77, 1983
16. Neer S II. Impingement syndrome revisited (orthopaedic transcript). Presented at the Interim Meeting of the American Orthopaedic Society for Sports Medicine, 8:70–71, 1984
17. Neer CS II, Marberry TA. On the disadvantages of radical acromionectomy. J Bone Joint Surg [Am] 63:416–419, 1981

18. Neviaser TJ, Neviaser RJ. Lesions of long head of biceps tendon. In: American Academy of Orthopaedic Surgeons. Instructional Course Lectures, vol 30, pp 250–257. AAOS, Chicago, 1981

19. Norwood LA, Del Pizzo WJ, FW, Kerlan, RK. Anterior shoulder pain in baseball pitchers. Am J Sports Med 6:103–106, 1978

20. Penny JN, Welsh RP. Shoulder impingement syndrome in athletes and their surgical management. Am J Sports Med 9:11–15, 1981

21. Perry J. Anatomy and biomechanics of the shoulder in throwing, swimming, gymnastics, and tennis. Clinics in Sports Medicine 2:247–270, 1983

22. Pujadas GM. Coracoacromial ligament syndrome. J Bone Joint Surg [Am] 52:1261–1262, 1970

23. Rathbun JB, MacNab I. The microvascular pattern of the rotator cuff. J Bone Joint Surg [Br] 52:540–553, 1970

24. Slatis P, Aalto K. Medial dislocation of the tendon of the long head of the biceps brachii. Acta Orthop Scand 50:73–77, 1979

25. Strizak A, Danzig L, Jackson D, et al. Subacromial bursography. J Bone Joint Surg [Am] 64:196–201, 1982

Evaluation and Treatment of Early-Stage Impingement Syndrome of the Shoulder in the Athlete

7

Frank W. Jobe
Benjamin Ling

Impingement of the shoulder is common in sports like swimming and baseball pitching that demand repetitive overhead motion. Neer (9) has demonstrated that the anterior acromion, coracoacromial ligament, and at times the acromioclavicular joint are the structures against which the rotator cuff and subacromial bursa impinge. He has also presented a staging system to aid in managing this problem (10).

Our experience with athletes under 35 years of age has led us to expand Neer's staging system to include the pathological progression found in this group. This staging system helps us establish the prognosis in these athletes. Stage I is that of edema and swelling of the rotator cuff; stage II is that of fibrosis and tendonitis, and can have some associated fiber disruption, including incomplete defects in the rotator cuff; stage III lesions are complete tears of the rotator cuff up to 1 cm in dimension; and stage IV lesions are greater than 1 cm in size. We have found that patients with stage IV lesions have a very poor prognosis for return to the previous level of overhead activity, particularly in the area of stamina. Stage III has a guarded prognosis for return to the previous level of performance in throwers and a bleak prognosis in swimmers. Stages I and II are usually reversible with proper selective rest and rehabilitation (6). This chapter will concentrate on the evaluation and treatment of stage I, II, and early stage III lesions. From the outset, we emphasize that the best treatment is prevention. Improper warm-up or warm-down, inadequate flexibility, muscular imbalance, strength deficits, overtraining, inadequate rest periods, and improper technique can all predispose the athlete to the development of an impingement syndrome. A properly designed and implemented conditioning and competitive program, individualized and monitored

65

to stay within the individual capacity for recovery, will help minimize the frequency and extent of this problem.

Clinical Presentation

The usual presentation is that of shoulder pain. The pain is often poorly localized and reported as deep inside. The complaint of night pain and difficulty lying on the involved shoulder is often present. The pain is made worse by activity of the arm in the overhead position. Neurological symptoms and symptoms of instability are absent unless there is a concurrent problem. The history should include a picture of repetitive use of the arm in the overhead position. Often closer questioning will bring to light obvious errors in training. Initially, the pain is made better with rest and is brought on with activity. As the syndrome progresses, a more constant pain can be present.

In the physical exam the examiner should look for subtle atrophy of the shoulder musculature. A careful measure of the range of motion of the involved

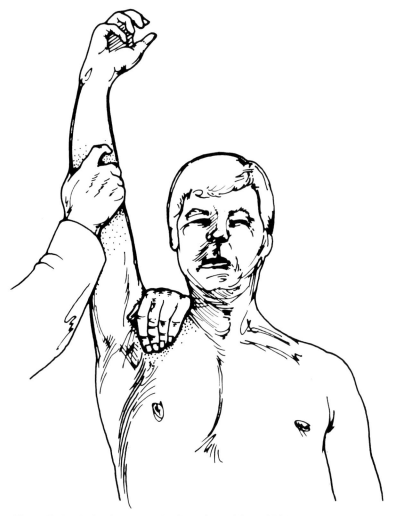

Figure 7-1 The impingement sign is performed by stabilizing the scapula with one hand while flexing the arm with the other hand in an effort to pinch the impinging structures.

and noninvolved extremity should be recorded. One should be reminded that in throwers the range of the dominant extremity can be significantly greater than that of the nondominant one; thus symmetrical range of motion can be abnormal at times. Careful palpation of the rotator cuff, biceps, acromioclavicular joint, and the anterior and posterior capsules should be performed. A screening neurological and circulatory exam should be included in every shoulder work-up. The impingement signs and tests as described by Neer (9) (Figure 7–1) and Hawkins and Kennedy (4) are helpful. We have frequently found the supraspinatus test positive (6). A bicipital tendonitis is often part of the syndrome complex. One should be sure to test for anterior, inferior, and posterior instability, which can have a presentation similar to an impingement problem. It is commonly informative to have the patient show the motion(s) and arm position(s) that give the most difficulty. Adding manual resistance as the patient goes through the motion slowly can be evocative.

In most instances a careful history and physical examination will make the diagnosis clear. On occasion it may be necessary to bring the athlete back for an additional visit or visits to allow for a more comprehensive or relaxed exam.

Ancillary Tests

We routinely get an anteroposterior roentgenogram of the shoulder, including the ipsilateral hemithorax as advocated by Rowe (11), an internal rotation view, and an axillary view. The hemithorax view is important to help avoid missing a neoplasm or associated pulmonary process.

If there is a high index of suspicion of a possible rotator cuff tear, we will order a double-contrast arthrogram (2), which we feel is more sensitive than single-contrast studies for detecting incomplete tears. Arthrotomography is useful in evaluation of labral lesions (3, 8). Bone scanning can be helpful to rule out avascular necrosis or neoplastic processes. Arthroscopy can be useful in particularly puzzling cases (1, 7).

Conservative Treatment

As previously stated, the best treatment is prevention. Our initial approach to those who do develop an impingement syndrome and do not have a documented tear is a prolonged conservative regimen. With rare exceptions, even those who have had a prolonged conservative course elsewhere will be required to undergo a closely monitored program of conservative care in our hands before we will consider surgical intervention. We consider 9–12 months a reasonable time period for conservative care. Our program of conservative care starts with a period of selective rest. This means avoiding aggravating activities until the inflammation is under control while maintaining general body conditioning. In addition to selective rest, we use an anti-inflammatory, flexibility, and strengthening program. Our anti-inflammatory program includes oral anti-inflammatory medication, ice, and electrical stimulation. On occasion, we will use an injection of dilute steroid to help break the inflammatory cycle. Any muscle imbalances or deficits should be identified and corrected. A functional range of motion must be maintained or achieved. If the athlete remains symptomatic, we will then consider surgical intervention. If the athlete is a swimmer, he or she should be made aware that the chances of returning to the previous competitive level are minute. For those involved in other overhead sports, the prognosis is guarded. Unrestrained optimism may pave the way for marked disappointment.

Operative Treatment

In those patients who have a documented complete tear, we recommend early operative intervention and repair. A prolonged conservative program may allow a stage III lesion to progress to stage IV. When treating those with stage I and II lesions that fail to respond to a reasonable conservative program, we present the option of surgery or an extension of the conservative program. It is not clear at this time whether those that undergo surgical management with an acceptable result would have responded just as well to an extended conservative program. The final decision must be made in conjunction with the athlete; both physician and patient must take into consideration future demands and aspirations.

Although some have had good success with resection of the coracoacromial ligament for recalcitrant impingement syndromes (4, 5), we have not found this to be a satisfactory procedure in our hands. We have had more success with partial acromioplasty combined with resection of the coracoacromial ligament, done in a manner similar to that described by Neer (9).

The patient is placed in the lateral decubitus position (Figure 7–2) and supported firmly with a Vacu-Pak (Olympic Medical, Seattle, WA). A kidney rest posteriorly may be helpful. Care should be taken to have the axilla properly free, to pad adequately the bony prominences in the lower extremity, and to have the peroneal nerve free as it courses around the neck of the fibula.

An 8-cm saber-type incision is made midway between the acromioclavicular joint and the lateral tip of the acromion (Figure 7–2). The skin flaps are then undermined for visualization. The raphe between the anterior and middle thirds of the deltoid is identified and carefully incised for a distance of about 3–4 cm from the acromion (Figure 7–3). Care should be taken to avoid incising the underlying rotator cuff. As the edges of the incision are lifted, the anterior and middle portions

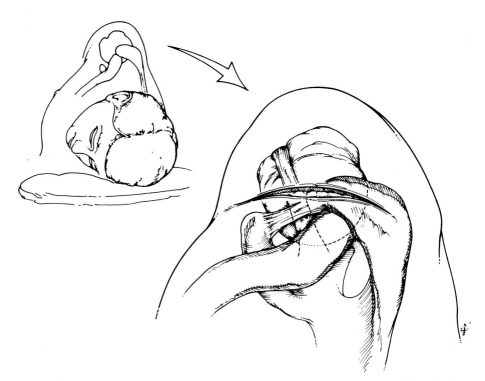

Figure 7–2 With the patient in the lateral decubitus position, a saber incision is made.

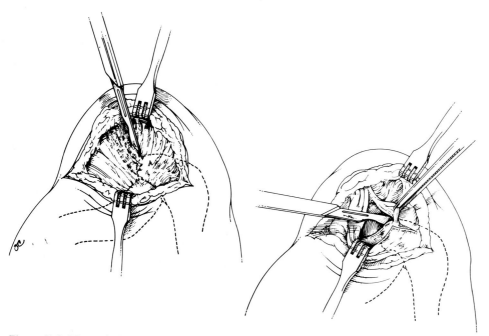

Figure 7–3 The raphe between the anterior and midportions of the deltoid is identified and incised. The deltoid is elevated as described in the text.

of the deltoid are carefully dissected from the acromion for a distance of about 1.5 cm in the direction of the middle third and 2 cm in the direction of the anterior third (Figure 7–3). An attempt should be made to take as much of the periosteum with the deltoid flaps as possible to facilitate better reattachment. The deltoid is freed from the underlying subacromial bursa. If the bursa is thickened and inflamed, we remove the portion that is accessible. Rotation of the arm will help in exposure of the bursa.

Once good exposure is obtained, we use a ¾-inch curved osteotome to perform a partial acromioplasty. We attempt to remove the anterior one-third of the undersurface of the acromion (Figure 7–4). Usually we are able to remove part of

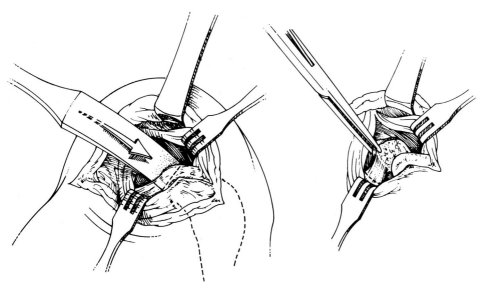

Figure 7–4 A curved osteotome is used to do the initial partial acromioplasty.

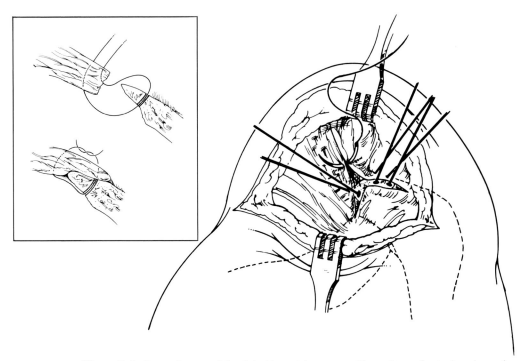

Figure 7–5 Reattachment of the deltoid must be secure. The pattern of suturing shown in the inset brings the deltoid above the acromion, thus preventing an iatrogenic impingement.

the coracoacromial ligament along with the acromioplasty. What remains of the ligament is sharply resected. A rongeur is used to "fine tune" the acromioplasty. We would much rather remove too little bone than too much with the initial cut, to minimize the risk of acromial fracture. Once the acromioplasty and ligament resection are completed, we palpate the undersurface of the acromion and carefully bring the arm into the impingement position. If there are any bony spikes or if the decompression seems inadequate, we then take more bone with the rongeur. The rotator cuff and biceps tendon are inspected at this time. Any thinning and inflammation is noted. The wound is then irrigated and closed. The most important step of closure is proper reattachment of the deltoid to the acromion. The deltoid must be securely refastened to the acromion and in such a way that it will not in itself become part of an impingement process. We use no. 0 nonabsorbable suture in a loop configuration (Figure 7–5). Usually three of these sutures are sufficient, and the closure of the deltoid is then augmented with some absorbable suture. The subcutaneous layer is closed with absorbable suture and the skin is closed with a subcuticular suture. This is reinforced with skin tapes. The patient is placed in a sling postoperatively.

Rehabilitation

The patient is started on gentle passive abduction and external rotation exercises on the first postoperative day. There are continued at home for 1 month. Active assisted exercises are initiated in the second month. After the deltoid is secure at 9 weeks, a more aggressive rehabilitation program can be started. This includes active range of motion, stretching exercises, and careful strengthening. Once full range of motion has been obtained, a graduated return to activity can be planned. The rehabilitation program must be carefully monitored by the treating physician and modified according to patient response.

Summary

1. Prevention is the best treatment of impingement syndrome.
2. Most of those with stage I and II lesions will respond to a conservative program.
3. A surgical approach is presented for those unresponsive to conservative care.
4. The prognosis for return to the previous level of competition is guarded in cases of operative intervention, particularly in swimmers.

References

1. Andrews JR, Carson WG, Ortega K. Arthroscopy of the shoulder: Technique and normal anatomy. Am J Sports Med 12:1–7, 1984
2. Berman JL, Shaub MS. Arthrography of the shoulder. Clinics in Sports Medicine 2:291–308, 1983
3. El Khoury GY, Albright JR, Abu Yousef MM, et al. Arthrotomography of the glenoid labrum. Radiology 131:333–337, 1979
4. Hawkins RJ, Kennedy JC. Impingement syndrome in athletes. Am J Sports Med 8:151–158, 1980
5. Jackson DW. Chronic rotator cuff impingement in the throwing athlete. Orthop Trans 1:24, 1977
6. Jobe FW, Moynes DR. Delineation of diagnostic criteria and a rehabilitation program for rotator cuff injuries. Am J Sports Med 10:336–339, 1982
7. Lombardo SJ. Arthroscopy of the shoulder. Clinics in Sports Medicine 2:309–318, 1983
8. McGlynn FJ, El Khoury GY, Albright JP. Arthrotomography of the glenoid labrum in shoulder instability. J Bone Joint Surg [Am] 64:506–518, 1982
9. Neer CS II. Impingement lesions. Clin Orthop 173:70–77, 1983
10. Neer CS II, Welsh RP. The shoulder in sports. Orthop Clin North Am 8:583–591, 1977
11. Rowe C. How I assess the shoulder, or "tricks of the trade," emphasis on hockey. Paper Presented at the American Academy of Orthopaedic Surgeons meeting on the Shoulder in the Athlete. Los Angeles, 1983

Surgical Considerations for Rotator Cuff Tears in Athletes

8

Russell F. Warren

Rotator cuff tears are generally the result of attritional changes occurring in the cuff over a period of years. Generally these occur in the late 50s as a result of minimal trauma disrupting a weakened tendon that has already undergone degeneration over a period of years. Usually this affects the supraspinatus initially, starting at the area of decreased vascularity just proximal to the greater tuberosity (Figure 8–1). Often these patients have had a history of "bursitis" intermittently for years. In the athlete the time course and age of presentation are markedly accelerated. In the population at large, cuff tears are extremely rare before age 30, but in athletes in certain sports, they may occur at an early age in either a slow progressive fashion, secondary to the microtrauma of overuse, or acutely, secondary to a single major injury.

It appears that the impingement syndrome is frequently a precursor to rotator cuff disruption, and as such, participants in the throwing sports are the most susceptible to cuff tears. This would include in particular baseball and tennis, and any sport utilizing the overhead position. Although swimmers have a high incidence of shoulder pain, it is uncommon for this to progress to a cuff tear since most swimmers decrease their activity significantly after 20–25 years of age. Perhaps with the masters athletic program we will see more cuff tears in swimmers. However, rotator cuff inflammation is a significant problem, as well as the progressive development of shoulder instability and labrum damage. Swimmers often practice 7,000–20,000 yards/day, and to do this, complete a stroke in 0.6 sec, traveling 1.9 m/sec (1). Thus, with this type of repetitive load, the rotator cuff is stressed considerably.

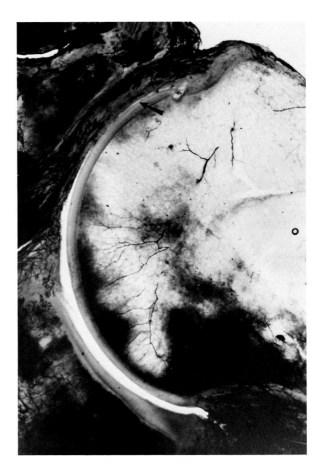

Figure 8–1 Injection study of shoulder cuff vascularity demonstrating relatively poor filling of rotator cuff proximal to the greater tuberosity (study by Steven Arnoczky and Russel F. Warren).

In baseball the rotator cuff will be active at varying times in the sequence of throwing. During the cocking phase, a torque of 17,000 kg/cm is generated (2). The wind-up phase is performed mainly by the deltoid, while the cocking phase is concluded by the activation of the subscapularis and pectoralis major. During the acceleration phase the rotator cuff, in skilled athletes, is quiet, but in unskilled individuals it may fire. The follow-through phase will activate the infraspinatus and teres minor to decelerate the humeral head (3). This activity performed repeatedly over time subjects the rotator cuff to high forces with resulting strain. As a result inflammation associated with swelling may compromise the subacromial space, resulting in an impingement syndrome (Figure 8–2). Although this will not generally produce a cuff tear in the high school athlete, it may in the college or professional athlete with the continued activity of throwing.

A similar mechanism occurs in tennis, again with the impingement problem frequently occurring. In contrast to baseball, tennis will be played by many patients into an age period in which rotator cuff degeneration commonly develops. Thus the physician will be confronted by many 40- to 50-year-old tennis players with a painful shoulder, in whom an impingement syndrome has progressed to a torn rotator cuff.

A second situation in which a cuff tear will be seen in the athlete is when a significant injury has occurred. This may or may not be associated with a dislocation. Dislocation occurring after age 40 will have a high incidence of rotator cuff tears, and it should be considered in young patients if pain persists for 2–3 weeks after a dislocation. We have seen this occur in football following a tackle that resulted in a dislocation. We have seen a number of skiers over a wide age range

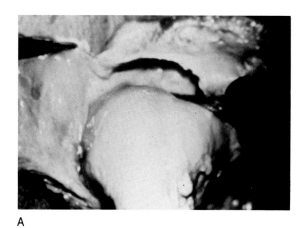
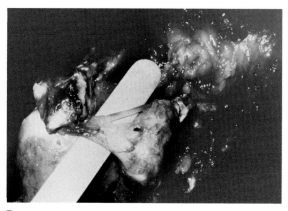

A   B

Figure 8–2 A Subacromial space demonstrates the edge of the coracoacromial ligament and its relationship to the rotator cuff and biceps tendon (arrow). **B** The coracoacromial ligament, viewed from above, demonstrating its Y configurement.

present with a rotator cuff tear following a fall. In some a dislocation occurred, whereas in others the force was high enough to disrupt the rotator cuff. In young patients this tends to be an avulsion injury, whereas in patients in their 50s, the tear occurs in an attenuated portion of the supraspinatus. In other patients tears may occur following injections for tendonitis after which sports were resumed too rapidly, resulting in a tear of the weakened tendon. Thus in evaluating your patient, an awareness that a cuff tear, although uncommon, may occur in the young athlete is important. Young patients presenting in a slow progressive manner may not demonstrate significant weakness but only complain of pain. Many of the characteristic findings of cuff tears seen in the elderly will be absent in the athlete complaining mainly of pain during or after activity and perhaps some decrease in speed or power. In contrast, many of those presenting with an acute injury with or without a dislocation have marked weakness on abduction secondary to the avulsion of the cuff. A second diagnostic possibility to consider in this situation is that of a brachial plexus injury involving the C5–C6 roots or the axillary nerve, which can closely mimic the weakness of a rotator cuff tear. In some of these patients, the sensation may remain intact, yet the motor function is markedly diminished. In evaluating these patients an arthrogram is obtained initially to rule out a cuff tear, followed by electromyograms at 2½–3 weeks if the arthrogram is negative and nerve damage is still suspected (Figure 8–3).

To evaluate the size of the rotator cuff tear, the use of tomograms combined with arthrograms may provide some insight. However, a useful clinical sign is the loss of power of the external rotators. Testing for the strength of the external rotators is important since weakness will indicate an extension of a tear posteriorly along the greater tuberosity, involving the infraspinatus.

Arthroscopy

Arthroscopy is playing a larger role in the evaluation and treatment of the painful shoulder in the athlete. Arthrograms may be negative, yet significant intraarticular pathology is present including labral tears, partial thickness rotator cuff tears, and biceps lesions. Since the results of open surgery in the throwing athlete are often less than satisfactory, we have increasingly utilized arthroscopic surgery in this population. Regarding rotator cuff lesions, partial thickness tears may be seen in

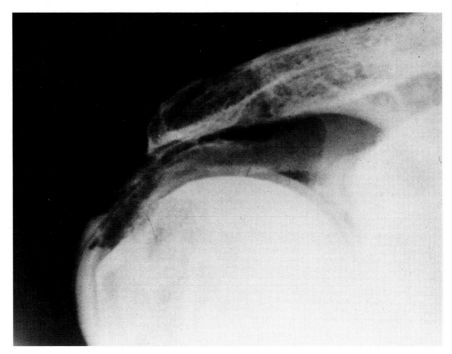

Figure 8–3 Arthrogram demonstrating dye within the deltoid bursa after a tear of the rotator cuff.

surprisingly young patients where fronds of tissue result in painful throwing. Debridement of this tissue may alleviate their pain allowing them to throw, although over time progression of their condition may occur. However, in selected patients this is an alternative to open surgery. In young active patients with partial tears, demonstrated by arthrograms, a conservative approach utilizing spring or elastic exercises to develop the rotator cuff would be appropriate initially, followed by arthroscopy if pain persisted. In those patients with a documented full thickness tear a more aggressive approach is indicated, particularly if this is the result of an acute injury in contrast to a slowly progressive condition.

Operative Approach

We will explore the rotator cuff by utilizing a superior approach that allows for an acromioplasty to be performed. The incision will run along the outer edge of the acromion to the coracoid process (Figure 8–4, A). The deltoid is partially detached anteriorly from the acromion to the acrommioclavicular (AC) joint. A longitudinal split is made within the deltoid fibers distally for 4–5 cm (Figure 8–4, B). Further dissection is not possible because the axillary nerve will be encountered. Generally, the deltoid is detached slightly obliquely to leave some soft tissue on the acromion. Next the inferior surface of the acromion is exposed and all soft tissue attachments are removed. An acromioplasty is generally performed at the time of cuff repair since the impingement process has played a role prior to the tear in older patients, and in younger patients with an avulsion type of injury, the cuff will thicken during the repair process, increasing the compression in this region. Thus an acromioplasty generally will be a component of the repair procedure. In addition, it will improve your visualization of the cuff tear. To perform the acromioplasty, a sharp osteotome is placed at the edge of the anterior acromion after dissecting off the soft tissue. The osteotome is angled to avoid the AC joint. The portion of bone to be removed consists of the inferior aspect of the anterior half of the acromion. When viewed from a lateral projection, the acromion has a concave appearance; thus the osteotome should be angled to exit the bone at the midpoint of the acromion. If the AC

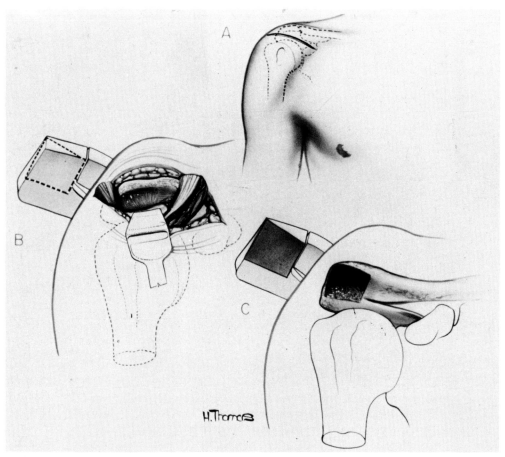

Figure 8–4 Acromioplasty. **A** Superior incision for acromioplasty or rotator cuff repair. **B** Outline of bone to be removed from anterior half of acromion. **C** In performing acromioplasty one attempts to avoid the acromioclavicular joint. If there are spurs under the joint, these may be smoothed off with a burr.

joint is prominent inferiorly, then the spurs are removed using a burr, but the joint is preserved unless there is significant degenerative arthritis that is felt to be causing symptoms. The bursa is partially excised since it is often thickened and inflamed, further compromising the subacromial space.

The rotator cuff tear is then identified. These are graded as to size: <2 cm in length represents a small tear; 2–5 cm, a moderate tear; and >5 cm, a large tear. In the athletic population in which the injury is a result of overuse, the tear will generally be in the small range. Conversely, when there is significant trauma involved in a young athlete, then a large tear of the avulsion type will be seen at the attachment site instead of slightly proximal in the poorly vascularized area. In an older athlete the tear may represent significant trauma superimposed on a degenerating tendon. In this situation the tear may be large but will occur in the more typical area of decreased vascularity at the site of previous degeneration (Figure 8–1).

In performing a repair of the rotator cuff certain principles are important:

1. Obtain good visualization of the defect.
2. Adequately decompress the subacromial space.
3. Perform an adequate release of the rotator tendons to allow repair without tension. This includes releasing outside the tendon as well as within the joint in large tears.

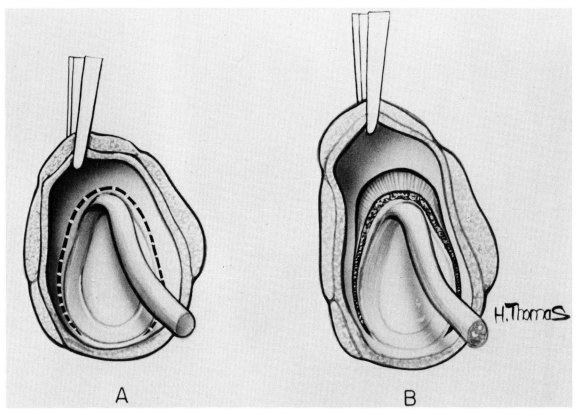

Figure 8–5 Relaxing incision of capsular attachment to labrum may be necessary if rotator cuff tear has become fixed in a retracted position. Release combined with lysis of superficial adhesions will allow even long-standing tears to be advanced.

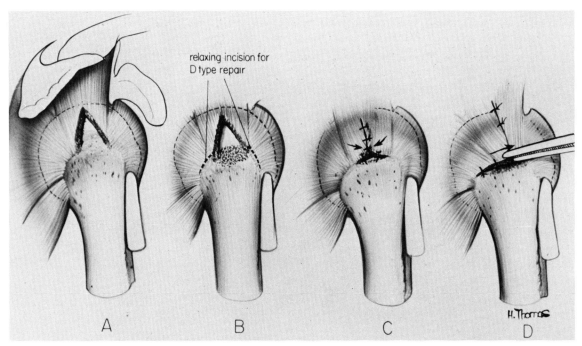

Figure 8–6 **A** Relatively small tear (less than 2 cm in long axis), which afterwards will form a V shape as the supraspinatus retracts. **B** Preparation of bony bed to receive tendon. This area is roughened to bleeding bone and is made as broad as possible to promote tendon reattachment. **C** V tear may be converted to partial Y and advanced laterally with or without relaxing incision. **D** If V tear is long and difficult to close, one edge may be advanced to fill defect hinging on apex of tear. This will require a relaxing incision.

4. Provide a broad, bleeding, bony surface for attachment of the tendons as the rotator cuff itself will be relatively avascular at the site of the tear.
5. Avoid tenodesing the biceps tendon or using it in the repair unless the tendon is grossly inflamed, unstable, or necessary to aid the repair in large tears.
6. Reattach the cuff with nonabsorbable sutures without tension.
7. Utilize a splint for all moderate and large tears.
8. Start early passive motion in safe ranges determined at surgery.

In performing a repair, I will initially place retention sutures in the tendon to allow traction to be placed on the cuff. To restore the correct length to the tendon, dissection is performed outside of the tendons initially and subsequently within the joint, on larger long-standing tears, when the tendons have retracted. In degenerated lesions in younger patients the tear will generally be small unless trauma played a major role in the etiology. In such cases correction of the impingement process is the major goal of surgery. If a tear is moderate or large, then an aggressive approach to restore the length of the retracted tendon is necessary. This is accomplished by dissecting within the joint to separate the contracted capsule from the tendon just peripheral to the labrum (Figure 8–5). In freeing the tendon a judgment is made as to the ability to advance the torn cuff to a bony bed. Often the retraction of the tendons has made a straight tear into a V or a rectangle. This will require a Z-plasty to be performed to reattach the tendons and avoid a bulge in the tendon (Figure 8–6). If an overlap is created in advancing the tendon, then a portion may be excised (Figure 8–6, D).

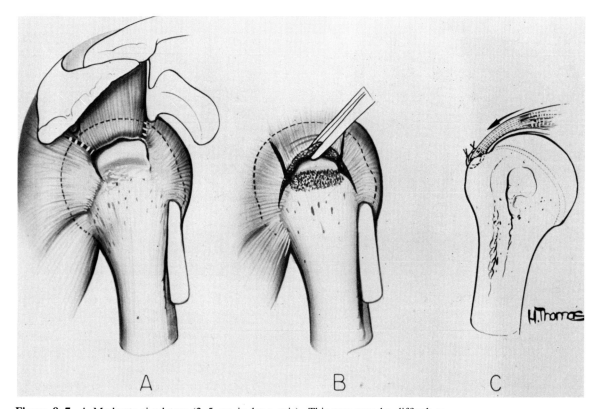

Figure 8–7 **A** Moderate-sized tear (2–5 cm in long axis). This tear may be difficult to close and may require extensive dissection on both sides of rotator cuff. **B** Relaxing incisions parallel to fibers of cuff to coracoid and spine of scapula may be required to advance retracted segment. This is combined with capsular release. **C** Tendon is advanced to bone bed and attached with nonabsorbable sutures placed through the cortex.

In preparing the bony bed, a broad surface is created to provide an extensive bleeding surface for fibrous ingrowth. This will be from the edge of the articular surface to the tuberosity (Figure 8–7). The lateral cortical bone is spared to facilitate a firm attachment site unless an overgrowth of the tuberosity is a component of the impingement process. In this case it is trimmed initially.

Subsequently, if a V-type tear is present, the repair is performed in a proximal to distal fashion utilizing nonabsorbable sutures. The edge of the tendon is advanced to the prepared bone and sutured in place over a broad area, with a mattress suture through the lateral cortex of the tuberosity (see Figure 8–7).

Large tears will require some imagination from the surgeon when performing the repair. Large contracted tears will be unusual in the younger athlete, but in middle-aged to older patients, large tears may be encountered that will severely test one's abilities. At times we have been confronted by a 65- to 75-year-old tennis player who enjoys tennis 5–6 days a week and has noticed a loss of power. The x-rays demonstrate marked superior migration of the humeral head consistent with a massive tear. In this situation a conservative approach is best, as you can easily make this patient worse. In general, I feel that pain relief can be achieved with a considerable degree of predictability, but strength improvements are dependent on the quality of the soft tissues as well as one's abilities to perform a repair.

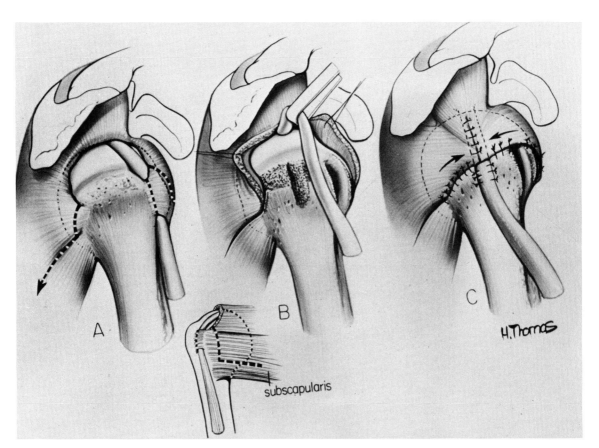

Figure 8–8 **A** Large (longer than 5 cm in long axis) rotator cuff tear. To close this defect, cuff must be released posteriorly, freeing infraspinatus from the teres minor. Anteriorly, subscapularis is incised at junction of the lower third. **B** Repositioning of biceps tendon into more posteriorly positioned groove to aid closure of defect. **C** Superior advancement of infraspinatus and subscapularis to biceps tendon. This leaves a defect anteriorly and posteriorly.

If surgery is attempted in a massive tear, an aggressive mobilization of the cuff is critical (Figure 8–8). The attempt is to advance the cuff distally to cover the humeral head to establish a fulcrum for humeral head elevation. Incorporation of a component of the biceps may be necessary. These large, degenerated tears are not generally seen in athletes, but are a function of long-standing attritional changes in advanced age. The extensive repairs necessary are not pertinent to the athletic population.

Rehabilitation

Following repair of the cuff, I feel that the use of a splint is important (Figure 8–9). A splint will allow the tendons to heal in a relaxed position. In addition, there is some suggestion that the vascularity of the cuff in this region is improved by some abduction (4). Probably of more importance is a passive exercise program that may be initiated from the splint in arcs that are determined at surgery so as not to stress the repair. Thus passive forward flexion to 90 degrees and external rotation to 20 degrees may be started several days after surgery when some of the initial soft tissue swelling is receding. It is my impression that improved continuous passive motion machines will aid in this approach.

Generally, the approach to therapy will be guided by the size of the tear, the quality of the tissue, and the ability to perform an adequate repair. Early motion may be initiated during the first week or held off for 4–6 weeks. In the younger active patient with good tissues, passive motion is started primarily at day 4–6 and progresses in safe ranges. A muscle stimulator is applied to the deltoid. After 4–6 weeks, active assisted movement is begun, progressing to fully active movement at 6 weeks. Following this, rotator cuff strengthening exercises are started. Therabam rubber tubing is utilized, followed by a spring exercise program initially performed at the side but progressing to the 90-degree abducted position over 6–8

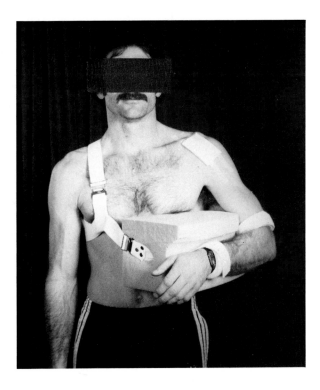

Figure 8–9 KW abduction splint utilized to decrease stress on the repaired tendons. Early passive motion may be initiated from the splint in selected arcs.

weeks. Light weights are then utilized in flexion, avoiding abduction, which tends to aggravate impingement symptoms. Nautilus activity may be started around 4–6 months postoperatively in a selected fashion.

Generally, throwing activities are avoided for about 9 months, but swimming may be started around 6 months. With this approach some success in returning to active sports can be achieved, but it is unlikely that an individual will return to a high level of throwing activity; rather, the improvement in pain and strength will allow resumption of sports activities at a lower level of performance in which skill instead of power is emphasized.

References

1. Counsilman JE. Forces in swimming: Two types of crawl stroke. Res Q 26:127–139, 1955
2. Freedman L, Munro RR. Abduction of the arm in the scapular plane: Scapular and glenohumeral movements. J Bone Joint Surg [Am] 48:1503–1510, 1966
3. Jobe FW, Tibone JE, Perry J, et al. An EMG analysis of the shoulder in throwing and pitching. Am J Sports Med 11:3–5, 1983
4. Rathbun JB, MacNab T. The microvascular patterns of the rotator cuff. J Bone Joint Surg [Br] 52:540, 1970

Arthroscopic Evaluation and Surgery for Rotator Cuff Disease

9

A.M. Wiley

The adaptation of the arthroscope to surgery of the shoulder is certainly a development of some significance. Surgeons will find it difficult to avoid comparing the future for arthroscopic shoulder surgery to that of the knee, which has been revolutionized by the arthroscope. Indeed, the prudent surgeon should be careful to avoid overuse of these instruments.

What has the arthroscope to offer, particularly for rotator cuff "disease?" We are talking abut rotator cuff tears, in essence.

Tendonitis is an ill-defined term. Calcification is frequently asymptomatic and easily diagnosed. Why arthroscope when good x-rays, arthrograms, and arthrotomograms are available to us? What has rotator cuff disease to do with athletes? Surely this is an elderly person's disease?

In spite of our methods, however, our cases often remain imprecisely diagnosed, labeled by such terms as "pitcher's shoulder," "swimmer's shoulder," "instability," "bursitis" and, of course, "tendonitis." While such terms may satisfy the surgeon, they are poor comfort to an athlete, especially a professional.

While Codman (1) and DePalma (2) described rotator cuff tears in fully one-third of cadavers, we are led to believe that the majority of them were, in life, symptomless. (In our own review of symptomatic tears of the rotator cuff, fully 20% were in patients below the age of 40 years.)

Even the best arthrograms fail to show partial tears of the rotator cuff. Most surgeons would agree now that the symptoms of smaller rotator cuff lesions are merely "impingement." Therefore, how can we exclude the rotator cuff tear in the swimmer, the ball player, and the tennis player? Although such an obvious lesion may be unlikely in the very young, this is not so in middle-aged and weekend athletes, and above all in the older professionals.

I have reviewed 506 shoulder arthroscopies and make this presentation to describe the use of the shoulder arthroscope for (1) diagnostic and (2) therapeutic purposes, with special reference to rotator cuff disease.

Diagnostic Technique

The technique of shoulder arthroscopy for a diagnosis will be described here. Later, the supplementary maneuvers involved in arthroscopic bimanual surgery will be discussed. Most arthroscopic procedures require a general anesthetic, particularly for shoulder procedures, because of the need for an assistant to distract and maneuver the joint during the examination. The procedure can be carried out under a local anesthetic, using Marcaine, but this restricts some of the maneuvers considered important in making a diagnosis. It is recommended that the instrument be introduced posteriorly, with the patient in a lateral sit-up position. The examiner will find it easiest to insert the arthroscope one thumb's breadth below the angle of the acromion while the assistant distracts the arm to open the joint (Figures 9–1 and 9–2). Some surgeons may elect to use a Buck's extension apparatus or similar traction device in place of an assistant, but there have been records of brachial plexus palsy attributable to this maneuver, and the use of an assistant to intermittently distract the arm appears to be safer. (The surgeon should avoid manipulating the arm forcibly before introducing the instrument; this may fill the joint with blood and debris and make the subsequent maneuvers more difficult.) Manipulations can wait until the arthroscopy is complete.

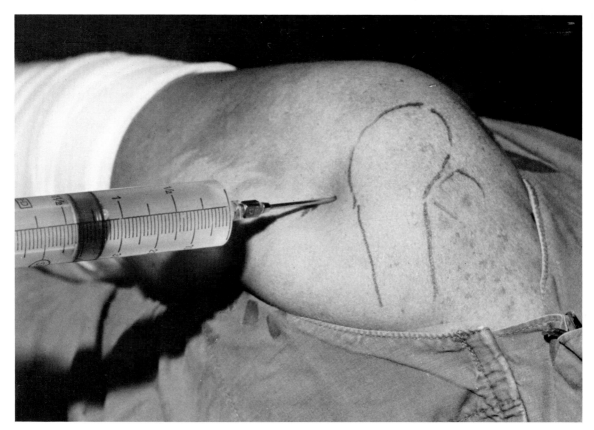

Figure 9–1 Distension of the shoulder prior to arthroscopy and point of entry for the instrument.

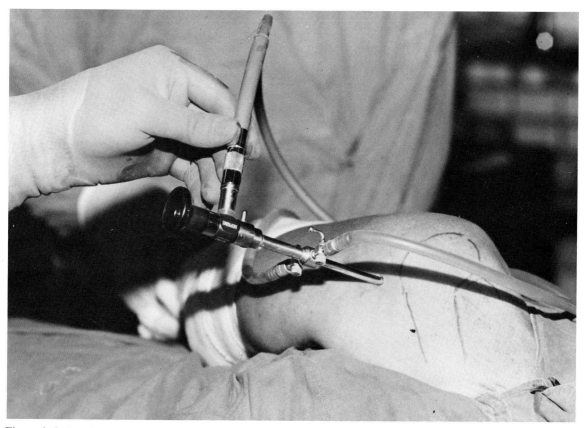

Figure 9–2 Introduction of arthroscope.

The joint is first distended with saline and its capacity is measured. The shoulder joint normally accepts 35 cc. Less than this may signify some element of frozen shoulder, and more than this is found in lax shoulders and in patients with significant rotator cuff tears. In cases subjected to previous operations, it is sometimes informative to culture the irrigate after the needle first enters the joint.

The examination of the shoulder should be conducted in an orderly fashion. First the surgeon locates the long head of the biceps, and in the supraglenoid region he will notice the rotator cuff shining through the synovial joint lining (Figure 9–3). It is usually possible to see the subscapularis, but there may be too thick a capsule to see this freely. The supraspinatus should be examined carefully, particularly at its insertion on the humeral head. The assistant should apply some abduction and distraction to enable the instrument to be inserted between the fibers of the insertion of the supraspinatus and the humeral tuberosity. By withdrawing the instrument one can examine the infraspinatus: an arthroscope with a 30-degree-angle lens is useful in this respect. Standard arthroscopes are perfectly satisfactory for the arthroscopic examination of the shoulder. The examiner then examines the middle or glenoid segment of the joint, looking particularly at the glenoid labrum anteriorly and posteriorly because disinsertion and flap tears of the labrum are quite common and may indicate instability. Indeed, these findings provide information about the direction of such instability, i.e., a posterior Bankart lesion will, of course, warn the examiner that the patient has posterior instability. Passing the instrument through to the front of the joint, the examiner will see the middle and inferior glenohumeral ligament. Usually above the middle glenohumeral ligament is the opening into the subcapsular bursa, and this may be blocked in cases of frozen shoulder. The instrument is then passed into the infraglenoid recess, where

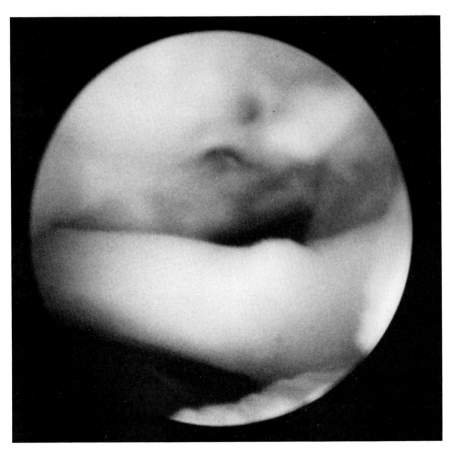

Figure 9–3 Arthroscopic appearance of the long head of the biceps, a reference point.

one may find loose bodies. This space is seldom obliterated. The examiner finally examines the humeral head while the assistant gently rotates the arm internally and externally, and this may reveal a Hill-Sachs lesion or degenerate changes on the humeral head. At the end of the shoulder arthroscopy the instrument is removed and it is at this stage that the examiner should test the shoulder for instability. A search should be made for multidirectional instability under these optimum conditions, with the patient anesthetized and the joint quite lax from the irrigation (Figure 9–4). In cases of indeterminate instability, the use of the image intensifier's C-arm may be helpful at this stage.

Examination of Tears of the Humeral Rotator Cuff

Complete and incomplete tears of the rotator cuff are readily seen by arthroscopy, and the accuracy of such examination seems to be quite high. In the author's experience with 15 cases of ruptured rotator cuff subsequently treated by open operation, the preoperative arthroscopy was accurate in 14. Although an arthrogram will assist the surgeon in the diagnosis of a complete rupture of the rotator cuff, arthroscopy can provide additional information. For example, arthroscopy can give a relatively accurate impression of the extent of the tear and its duration. Arthroscopy seems particularly indicated in patients suspected of having a rotator cuff tear but who were noted to have a negative arthrogram. Under these circumstances the arthroscopist can often detect an incomplete tear of the humeral rotator cuff. An additional investigation that is helpful under these circumstances consists of

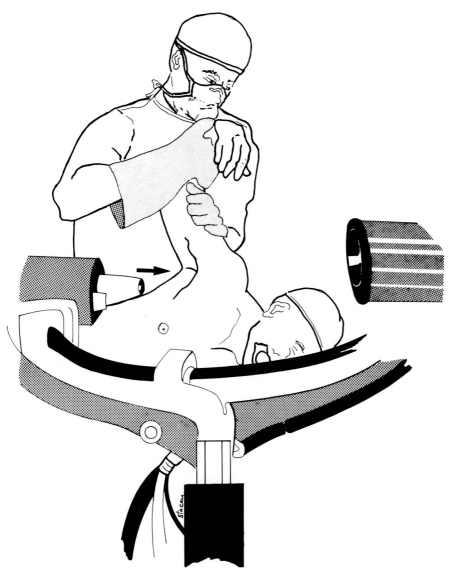

Figure 9–4 Manipulation of the shoulder after arthroscopy.

intraoperative arthrography. An infant's feeding catheter is passed along the sheath of the arthroscope, the telescope having been removed, and 30 cc of 60% Hypaque are instilled into the joint. An x-ray under these circumstances will give information about the integrity of the rotator cuff and whether a tear is complete or not. The number of incomplete tears that are seen in symptomatic shoulders is so high that it seems quite possible that the rotator cuff undergoes inevitable degeneration with splitting as the subject ages. The association of incomplete tears with the symptoms of impingement is common and will be referred to later. It is worth emphasizing that the rotator cuff is readily seen endoscopically with a 30-degree-angle lens in a standard arthroscope. The examiner should make a special effort to trace the insertion of the rotator cuff into the greater tuberosity to examine the biceps groove, and to withdraw and, if necessary, rotate the 30-degree-angle lens in an examination of the infraspinatus. It may be difficult to see clearly the subscapularis tendon anteriorly when the capsule and synovial lining are thickened, although tears of the subscapularis alone are, of course, rare.

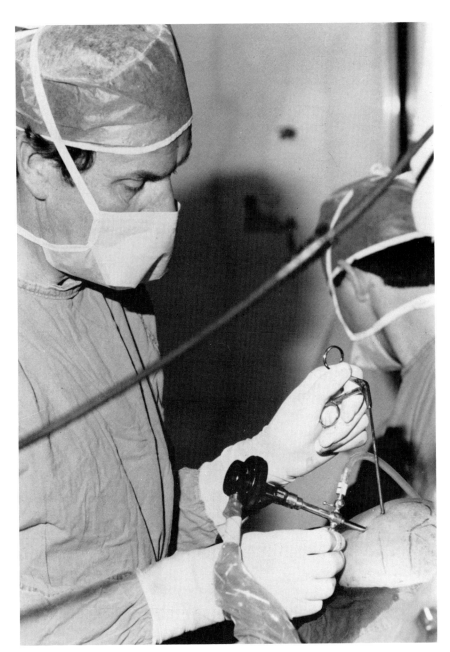

Figure 9–5 Posterior bimanual surgery.

Surgical Techniques

When the rotator cuff has been properly visualized and if it is found to be torn, either completely or incompletely, arthroscopic surgery may be performed.

Operating Arthroscopes

A 7-mm arthroscope is too large for free maneuvering within the shoulder. A 5-mm Storz arthroscope is provided with operating scissors and biopsy forceps

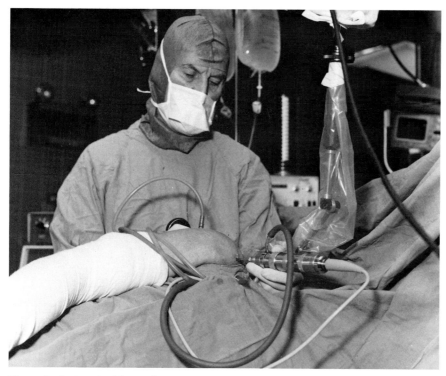

Figure 9–6 Anterior bimanual surgery.

that can be used together with 3.8-mm telescope. This equipment is useful for specific biopsies, limited debridement, and removal of loose bodies.

Bimanual Surgery Using a Posterior Route

Curved, 2.4-mm basket forceps or scissors may be introduced through the posterior route at a sufficient distance from the arthroscope to enable the surgeon's hand to maneuver the instruments into the shoulder. An entry is made into the posterior shoulder joint, using a sharp trocar. I usually use the sharp trocar provided with the Storz arthroscope sheath. This track may be followed by curved instruments—curved because of the contour of the humeral head. The 2.4-mm Wolff scissors or basket forceps is most useful for debriding the undersurface of the rotator cuff, removing suture material, and debriding the ragged edges of a torn rotator cuff (Figure 9–5).

Bimanual Surgery Using an Anterior Route

By shining the light of the arthroscope through the joint, the surgeon may find it relatively easy to insert a straight instrument into the front for direct visualization. This technique has been used for inserting the powered debriders and instruments. The instrument can be directed to the undersurface of the rotator cuff, and suction irrigation can be performed in this fashion (Figures 9–6 and 9–7).

It is emphasized that such debridement procedures are in each instance preceded by distension and irrigation and completed by a manipulation of the joint. The effect of the irrigation and manipulation may be of significance in assessing the results of this treatment. (See the following section.)

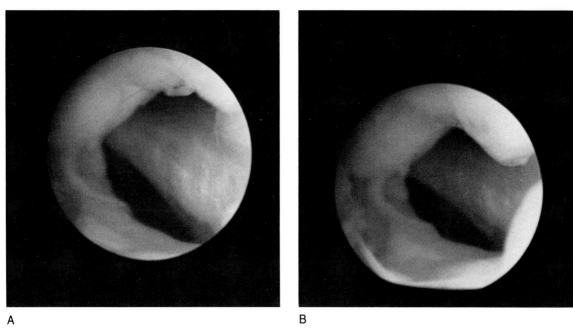

A   B

Figure 9-7 **A** Torn rotator cuff, edges already debrided. **B** Torn rotator cuff, alternate view. The coracoacromial ligament is seen crossing the subacromial bursa.

Case Selection for Arthroscopic Rotator Cuff Surgery

The role of the arthroscope in the diagnosis of rotator cuff disease may appear established. However, in the actual management of such conditions, the role of arthroscopic surgery must remain controversial, certainly until the results of such surgery are available from numerous surgeons in many centers, studying numerous cases over a lengthy period of time. A seasoned arthroscopist should have little difficulty in visualizing the rotator cuff, using standard instruments, and can just as easily learn to manipulate diseased areas. It is much more difficult to determine improvement and, if such improvement should occur, to attribute this to the instrumentation. For example, there is evidence of the beneficial effect of irrigation alone, especially with distension, on the shoulder afflicted with "pericapsulitis" [Lloyd et al. (3)], while manipulation is a technique long familiar to orthopaedists confronted with a stiff, painful shoulder. It would be appropriate to designate the irrigation of arthritic joints as a procedure for the "removal of prostaglandins." Orthopaedists, vexed with the natural history of rotator cuff disease, are confronted by patients with established tears fo the rotator cuff, who refuse treatment or undergo periods of physiotherapy, sometimes lengthy, and yet appear to make a satisfactory recovery. Evidence is available, however, to show that a shoulder afflicted with a complete tear of the rotator cuff never regains its full strength and frequently presents with episodic symptoms. The use of the Cybex has proved valuable in this respect and demonstrates impaired spinatus activity in chronic cases (W. A. Wallace, 1983, personal communication).

    The autopsy evidence that rotator cuff disease is common in the elderly is undeniable. Less certain is the belief that such subjects were symptomless. Indeed, more recent autopsy studies demonstrate a progressive deterioration in joints involved by rotator cuff disease, from tendinous tear to cartilage degeneration, ulceration, osteophytosis, eburnation, and subluxation. The recent work of Neer et al. (4) in describing the changes of ''rotator cuff arthropathy'' has confirmed the hazards to the shoulder joint surfaces in a shoulder affected by a torn rotator cuff. Symptomatic complete tears of the rotator cuff, therefore, justify a repair, as soon as possible after injury. Pain is the principal symptom in such cases, with stiffness, weakness, and impaired work ability being significant complaints. The results of such surgery are available in reviews of the literature.

Obviously, arthroscopic irrigation and debridement does not constitute a repair, yet I have been impressed by many patients who describe a relief of symptoms after this procedure. This is the same effect seen after debridement for the arthritic knee. The reasons for relief may lie in the irrigation, debridement, or distension. To be objective, for comparison purposes, we have used a series of our own of 18 cases, treated by open surgery for torn rotator cuff by the same surgeon (A.M.W.). All were treated with the same operative technique and were followed for 24 months. Fourteen patients were relieved of pain, 18 had return of useful movement, and 16 felt they could use the affected arm for work.

In a succeeding series of 20 patients treated for a complete rotator cuff tear by arthroscopic irrigation, debridement, and manipulation, after a follow-up period of 24 months, 16 were relieved of pain (5 completely, 11 relatively), 12 had improved range of movement, and 11 had returned to work. Two had retired and two were not employable for other reasons. The patient groups were similar in respect to age and sex. There was some bias towards adopting the arthroscopic technique for older patients, patients in whom the torn rotator cuff was an unexpected finding, and those who were ill-prepared for the rigors of a surgical repair followed by lengthy rehabilitation.

On the other hand, the outcome of arthroscopic debridement surgery in the treatment of incomplete tears of the rotator cuff was disappointing. Of 33 cases so treated, only 3 recovered, while 15 later underwent open decompression with excision of the meniscus or the acromioclavicular joint, complete resection of the coracoacromial ligament, and often, anterior acromioplasty. (The results of the open operation were excellent.)

Therefore, in the management of rotator cuff tears, arthroscopic surgery in the form of debridement and irrigation appears to be useful in treating chronic cases in older individuals. However, such treatment is inferior to routine subacromial decompression for patients suffering from the symptoms of impingement due to incomplete tears of the rotator cuff.

References

1. Codman EA. The Shoulder. Thomas Todd, Boston, 1934
2. DePalma AF. Surgery of the Shoulder, 3rd ed. JB Lippincott, Philadelphia, 1983
3. Lloyd GJ, Older MWJ, McIntyre JL. Distension arthroscopy of the shoulder joint. Can J Surg 19:203–227, 1976
4. Neer CS, Craig EV, Fukuda H. Cuff tear arthropathy. J Bone Joint Surg [Am] 65:1232–1247, 1983

Shoulder Replacement in the Athletic and Active Patient

10

Charles S. Neer, II
John J. Brems

Most surgeons would consider it inappropriate to discuss the use of any joint replacement in young, active, athletic people. Nevertheless, in the case of the shoulder, we have always recognized that a large proportion of the indications for replacement are in young adults and active middle-aged patients. These patients usually have good muscles and have the potential for achieving near-normal shoulder function following replacement. Fusions and resections make it impossible to use these muscles effectively, and for this reason such procedures are considered more radical than replacement, even in the younger age group. Fusions and resections are reserved for those with low-grade infection or with extensive destruction or paralysis of both the rotator cuff and deltoid muscles.

Since these active patients with good muscles have the potential for achieving near-normal function following shoulder replacement and have a very long life expectancy, it seems important to consider the precise indications, the type of replacement to be employed and its technique, the expectations for function, and the degree of activity compatible with the durability of the implant in this group of patients.

Indications in Active Patients

As shown in Table 10–1, of 500 recent shoulder replacements, 325 were performed in patients with severe trauma, avascular necrosis, arthritis of dislocations, and osteoarthritis. Patients with these conditions are often extremely active and have a very long life expectancy. Actually, it is striking to note that of the 500 shoulder

93

Table 10–1 Indications and Components Used for Shoulder Replacements in 500 Patients

	COMPONENT		
INDICATION	Humeral head	Total shoulder replacement	Fixed fulcrum
Trauma			
Acute	52		
Old	33	91	3
Avascular necrosis	19		
Osteoarthritis (primary and secondary)	6	89	
Arthritis of dislocation	2	30	
Rheumatoid arthritis	1	85	
"Elsewhere" prosthesis	3	43	
Cuff-tear arthropathy		25	
Miscellaneous (fusion, neoplasm, dysplasia, etc.)	4	14	—
	120	377	3

replacements, only 175 were done in patients with rheumatoid arthritis, cuff-tear arthropathy, neoplasms, and some of the other conditions that are found in inactive individuals. Patients with these conditions will not be considered in this discussion.

Trauma

Of the 179 patients who had shoulder replacements for severe fractures and fracture-dislocations with destruction of the humeral head, the average age was 54 years (1). The youngest was 14 years of age and approximately one-half were under 55 years of age. The injury was acute in 52 and over 6 months old in 127 patients. In those with acute injuries and in those with old injuries when the glenoid was in good condition, the humeral head component was used alone; however, a glenoid component was required in most of the old injuries. In this group of patients, the tuberosities were fractured and required accurate reduction and time for healing. This prolonged recovery, but when the muscles were normal, the eventual result was excellent. Most of the patients in this group were quite active and placed great demands on their shoulder (Figure 10–1). The fixed-fulcrum replacement used in three patients early in this series is no longer used.

Avascular Necrosis

Patients with steroid necrosis were usually under 35 years of age. The steroids had been given for a variety of diagnoses including thyroiditis, asthma, polymyositis, lupus, and spinal surgery. In a number of these patients, the initial medical diagnosis was later found to be an error, and the patient proved to be in good health with normal life expectancy. Many in this group were very athletic. Three patients, all under 30 years of age, were paraplegic and had received steroids at the time of their spinal injuries. These patients had bilateral humeral head necrosis, and since they used their arms for all transfers, their shoulders functioned like hip joints. Patients with infarctional diseases (such as sickle cell disease) were often young, and although they were not athletic, they often placed unusual loads on their shoulders because associated hip and knee involvement forced them to use

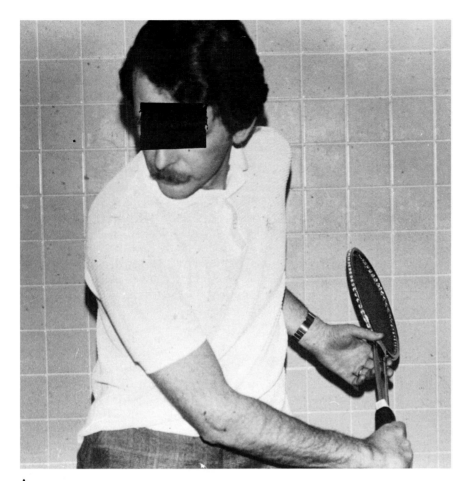

A

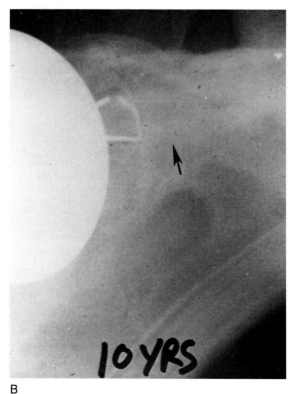

Figure 10–1 Ten-year followup of a standard polyethylene glenoid component in a high-level club tennis player who had been playing regularly four times a week since total shoulder replacement. **A** The patient whose right total shoulder had been done for a 9-year-old fracture with avascular necrosis and glenoid erosion. **B** Axillary view, made 19 years after fracture and 10 years after total shoulder replacement, showing no evidence of loosening or wear of the standard polyethylene glenoid component. The arrow indicates the bonecement interface.

B

crutches or canes. The humeral component alone was used in this group. When the necrotic humeral head had lead to glenoid erosion, requiring the glenoid component, the patient was classified with the secondary osteoarthritis category in Table 10–1.

Osteoarthritis

The 95 patients with osteoarthritis of the glenohumeral joint averaged 55 years of age (2). In this group of patients, the rotator cuff and deltoid muscles were intact, and typically, the patients were in the prime of life, healthy in all other respects, and had been actively engaged in tennis, golf, gardening, and other activities. One man who was 70 years old had been on the Davis Cup Tennis Team, but despite his love for tennis, had become unable to play. During the 7 years since the total replacement of his dominant shoulder, he has been playing tennis approximately 4 hours almost every day without apparent ill effects on the prosthesis. Several in this group play golf regularly, with an under 10 handicap. Eighty-nine patients in this group had nonconstrained total shoulder replacements, while 6 had humeral head replacement alone.

Arthritis of Dislocation

This is a newly recognized clinical entity (3). It is extremely important in sports medicine because most of the patients in this group have been extremely

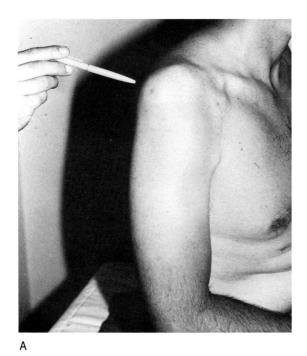
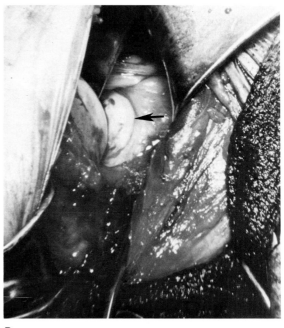

A   B

Figure 10–2. Arthritis of dislocations and the danger of doing a standard repair for recurrent anterior dislocations in an athlete who has multidirectional instability. **A** Preoperative photograph of a 38-year-old university coach and life-long athlete showing the scar anteriorly of a Putti-Platt procedure done 18 years previously that had tightened his anterior capsule, displacing the head into fixed posterior subluxation and leading to severe arthritis that required total shoulder replacement. Note the prominence of the coracoid, posterior alignment, and prominence of the humeral head, as in a posterior dislocation. **B** At surgery the head was found displaced backward, leaving the anterior glenoid empty (arrow) and causing deep erosion of the posterior glenoid, eburnation of the front of the head, and atrophy of the back of the head, requiring total shoulder replacement.

athletic. The majority had developed multidirectional dislocations (2) due to the stress of athletics (4) and had previous surgery for recurrent dislocations, which had tightened the anterior capsule and caused the head to be displaced posteriorly into the loose posterior pouch (Figure 10–2). The fixed posterior subluxation caused deep wear into the glenoid and destruction of the head. Although the average age of this group of patients was only 37 years, there was no good alternative to total shoulder replacement. The replacement procedure was particularly difficult because of scarring and weakness of the deltoid and shortening of the subscapularis from previous surgery, and the deep erosion of the glenoid, which often required a bone graft. Sports that most often lead to the arthritis of dislocations were football, weight lifting, and swimming. Although these patients are usually young, a glenoid component was used as well as a humeral component in all but 2 of the 32 (Table 10–1) because of the severe wear into the glenoid. As discussed in the section on technique and in Figure 10–3, we now prefer the recently released metal-backed

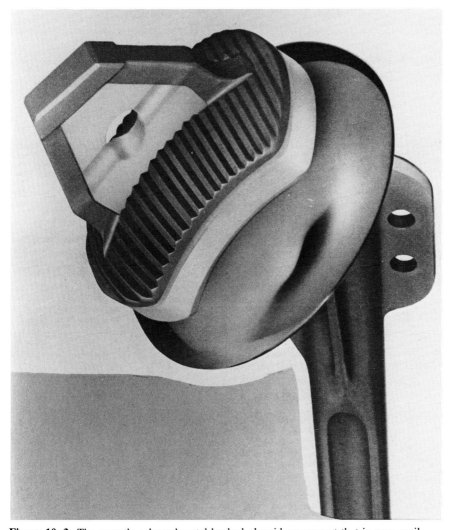

Figure 10–3 The recently released metal-backed glenoid component that is now available for general use and is preferred in active patients, especially when there has been wear and sloping of the glenoid. This component is anchored with acrylic cement. The humeral component is available with two lengths of head and a variety of stem sizes and can be used either with or without acrylic cement. The humeral component is used alone when there is a good glenoid, as in acute fractures and avascular necrosis.

glenoid component in this group. Special steps in the procedure include deltoid-plasty, lengthening of the subscapularis tendon, and not infrequently, a glenoid bone graft.

Technique of Replacement

As already discussed with each diagnostic category, each group presents special technical considerations in doing the procedure. However, the principle in all of our procedures is to preserve normal anatomy as much as possible, with minimal removal of bone, preservation of the muscles intact, and release of soft tissue adhesions. A meticulous postoperative rehabilitation program is considered essential. There would seem to be no place for a fixed-fulcrum, constrained prosthesis, especially in this active group of patients.

Regarding the implant used in this series, in 1973 the senior author revised the humeral component designed in 1951 so that the articular surface is no longer flattened on top. There are two lengths of head and the radius of curve of the articular surfaces of all components is 44 mm. This corresponds to the size of the average normal humeral head. Thirteen sizes of humeral components are available; of the nine glenoid components that have been used developmentally, two are now available for general use: the standard polyethylene component and the recently released, standard-sized, metal-backed unit. The metal-backed glenoid component (Figure 10–3) is preferred for active patients, especially when the glenoid is worn and sloping.

Although to date there has been no instance of reoperation required for loosening of the components, two polyethylene components have broken off in the scapula (leaving a portion firmly cemented within the scapula). Both of these complications occurred at about 2 years follow-up in very active patients who had had sloping glenoids. In both instances cement had broken out between the posterior part of the articular surface of the scapula and the polyethylene glenoid component. This allowed the polyethylene component to toggle until it finally fatigued and broke inside the bone. For this reason the metal-backed component is preferred in active patients, especially those with sloping glenoids.

The only approach used is the long deltopectoral approach, which leaves the origin of the deltoid entirely intact. Some of the anterior part of the deltoid insertion is often released to avoid too much trauma to the deltoid muscle during the procedure; however, this is carefully reattached at the end of the operation. This avoids the atrophy of the deltoid that occurs whenever the deltoid origin is taken down.

Patients with old trauma or the arthritis of dislocations in which the head has been subluxed or dislocated posteriorly for a long period of time often require special rehabilitation following nonconstrained replacement. Even though a posterior pouch has been closed at the time of the operation, the muscles are set for posterior displacement of the head. The exercise regimen must be directed at recovery of external rotation motion and strengthening of the external rotator muscles prior to subjecting the posterior capsule to stress. In these patients the humeral component is often placed in less than the usual amount of retroversion. In extreme cases of posterior instability, a spica with the arm in external rotation is used during the early postoperative period. In contrast, most patients with osteoarthritis and those with avascular necrosis have no problem with the muscles or instability, since the long deltopectoral approach leaves the muscles intact, these patients can be progressed from passive to active exercises by the 12th day following surgery.

Activities Permitted

With a properly implanted prosthetic unit and after rehabilitation of the muscles, these patients have been allowed virtually full activities except for impact loads (such as in contact sports and downhill skiing) and heavy weight lifting. They play tennis, golf, swim, and participate in basketball and in other noncontact recreational sports without restriction.

Some of these patients are unrealistic about body building and training. One man recently returned to follow-up saying that he had been lifting 250 pounds overhead and wanted to know if he could go further (Figure 10–4). He was promptly advised that overhead weight lifting was not permitted and that weights were limited to 50 pounds. Strengthening exercises below the horizontal using up to 50 pounds of resistance and push-ups are usually permitted. Overhead Nautilus exercises are not allowed.

Other activities such as gardening, farming, and construction work are performed by a number of these patients. They are advised to spare the shoulder by using the opposite arm for heavy lifting, by letting go of the hammer at the point of impact so the movement of the head of the hammer applies the force, and by using common sense.

Discussion

It has long been a surgical principle that any foreign objects or implant within a bone will eventually either break or loosen if it is subjected to sufficient pressure or stress. It would seem foolish to perform a joint replacement on any patient who is not willing to be realistic about the use of the implant. The senior author has refused to do joint replacements on a number of individuals who have seemed unwilling or unable to appreciate the need for some respect and precaution (Figure 10–4). An example of this is a weight lifter who refuses to give up heavy weight lifting or a professional stunt man who refuses to change his occupation. On the other hand, it does seem important to consider, in the light of our present knowledge and experience, what activities can be permitted a shoulder replacement in a reasonable patient.

During the period from 1953 to 1973 our patients used the press-fit humeral component (with a choice of five stem sizes and fenestrations for the ingrowth of bone) in virtually all activities including farming, carpentry, semiprofessional basketball, golf, and tennis without a problem of clinical loosening, provided the prosthesis had been firmly seated at the time of surgery. With the advent of the nonconstrained total shoulder replacement in 1973, it was thought that these new components used with and without acrylic cement should be subjected to the same stresses as their precursors to determine their durability and usefulness as compared to the humeral component alone. As shown in Table 10–1, we continue to use uncemented press-fit humeral components, especially when possible in younger patients, and have designed humeral and glenoid components with porous surfacing for developmental use without cement. It would seem desirable to use as little foreign material as possible, particularly in this active group. Nevertheless, we have not seen a problem of clinical loosening in our patients with this nonconstrained, cemented system, provided it has been properly installed; and, therefore, to date we see no reason to curtail the activities permitted. Since early active movement of the shoulder following replacement is essential to avoid adhesions, and the ingrowth of bone into cementless glenoid components requires a number of weeks, it is possible that the use of cementless glenoid components will introduce

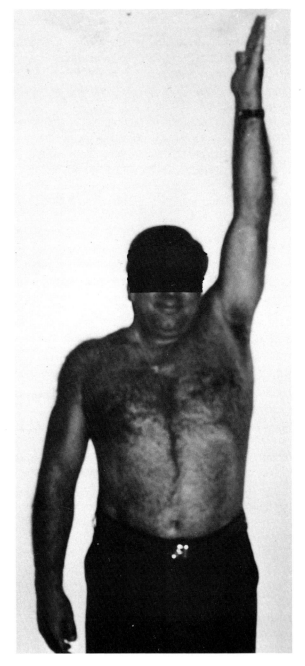

Figure 10–4 Despite a preoperative discussion about avoiding heavy, overhead weights after arthroplasty, at the regular follow-up 2 years after total shoulder replacement for osteoarthritis, this former weight lifter said he had resumed ''easy'' bench pressing of up to 250 pounds and wondered if he ''could go on up.'' He was promptly reminded of the preoperative discussion and again warned to stay under 50 pounds. Patients should be denied replacement arthroplasty if they are unwilling or unable to be realistic about the use of the implant. We allow noncontact sports, tennis, and golf but not heavy weight lifting or sports involving impact loads.

complications that we have not been seeing with the cemented units. In any event, it must be clear that we would not permit these activities unless the implant was soundly seated within the bone and stable (either with or without cement), the muscles had recovered tone and strength, and the patient had been made aware of the need for reasonable judgment and caution.

Summary

An effort has been made to discuss the indications for a nonconstrained shoulder arthroplasty in active patients and the activities allowed following this procedure.

Nonconstrained shoulder replacement is generally recognized as a technically difficult procedure because the reconstruction and rehabilitation of the muscles is more difficult than in other joints and is of equal importance to the seating and orientation of the components. Nevertheless, it is thought that a nonconstrained shoulder replacement, when properly inserted and designed to approach normal anatomy, has unique durability and function. Patients who are unwilling to confine their activities to reasonable levels are considered inappropriate for this procedure, however activities allowed following this replacement include noncontact sports, tennis, and golf. Heavy weight lifting and sports involving impact loads are not allowed.

References

1. Neer CS II. Fractures, Ed2 Chapter 11, Fractures about the shoulder. pp 675–707, Edited by CA Rockwood Jr. and DP Green, JB Lippincott, Philadelphia, 1984
2. Neer CS II. Replacement arthroplasty for glenohumeral osteoarthritis. J Bone Joint Surg [AM] 64:1–13, 1974
3. Neer CS II, Watson KC, Stanton FJ. Recent experience in total shoulder replacement. J Bone Joint Surg [AM] 64:319–337, 1982
4. Neer CS II, Foster CR. Inferior capsular shift for involuntary and multidirectional instability of the shoulder. A preliminary report. J Bone Joint Surg [AM] 62:897–908, 1980

Rehabilitation of the Shoulder

11

Andrew R. Einhorn
Douglas W. Jackson

Proper and individual shoulder rehabilitation will enhance both the nonoperative and operatively treated shoulder injury. It should begin as early as possible to minimize the effects of injury and shorten the period of disability. When properly done it may make a difference in whether or not an athlete can return to his or her chosen sporting activity.

Rotator cuff dysfunction has been recognized by many authors (1, 4, 5, 6, 9, 10, 11, 16, 19, 26, 27) as a particular challenge in the active person. Rehabilitating the athlete with a diagnosis of impingement syndrome associated with or withour rotator cuff injury should be conducted systematically and can be divided into three areas of concentration: decreasing inflammation, muscular and capsular stretching, and strengthening.

Decreasing Inflammation

Rest and rest alone from the aggravating activity is usually the most effective treatment of mild symptoms of inflammation in the athlete's shoulder. Rest is often too short. It may vary from a few days to months, depending upon the underlying injury and healing capabilities. During the rest phase, stretching and prevention of atrophy are started as soon as tolerated and within the limits of pain.

Several modalities are available to supplement the resolution of inflammation. Proper positioning of the shoulder enhances use of these modalities by exposing the specific portions of the rotator cuff. The patient, when seated with the shoulder internally rotated and adducted (Figure 11–1), moves the supraspinatus tendon out from under the anterior edge of the acromion. The posterior aspect of the rotator cuff can be made more accessible by external rotation and horizontal adduction (Figure 11–2). The posterior cuff muscles can be palpated just below the posterior acromion in this position. Figure 11–3 shows the patient receiving iontophoresis to the long head of the biceps. Placing the shoulder in extension causes the sub-acromial bursa to move anteriorly (8) (Figure 11–4). The patient is made to feel comfortable during all these treatments, and pillows can be used to help support the arm and shoulder.

A cardiovascular and muscular strengthening program during this phase of inflammation control is an integral part of sustaining the athlete's interest and enthusiasm. The general conditioning avoids any activity that will prolong or prevent healing. Riding a stationary bicycle and working the lower extremity muscle groups on weight equipment can usually be done without aggravating the impingement syndrome.

The swimmer emphasizes kicking until the shoulder pain decreases. The gymnast maintains strength and flexibility with selective routines that may not cause

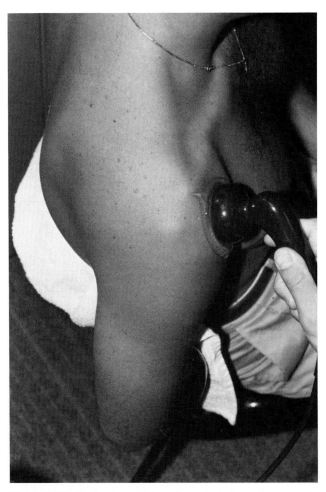

Figure 11–1 Patient is receiving phonophoresis to the supraspinatus tendon. Pulsed ultrasound may be used to avoid the thermal effects of ultrasound during the acute phase.

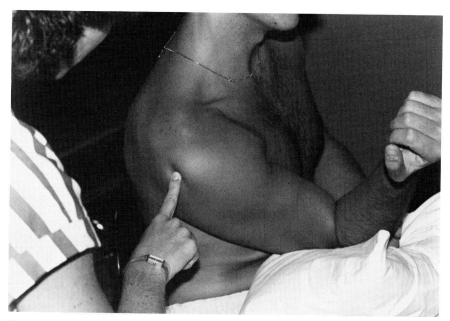

Figure 11–2 The posterior cuff is palpated (infraspinatus and teres minor). The athlete is positioned with the shoulder in horizontal adduction and external rotation.

symptoms. For example, in the case of ringman's shoulder, the rings are excluded and work is done on floor routines, forearm strengthening, and leg power exercises (27). It is important to develop an exercise program during the "rest phase" of rehabilitation so that when the athlete returns to his or her activity level, only the shoulder is the limiting factor.

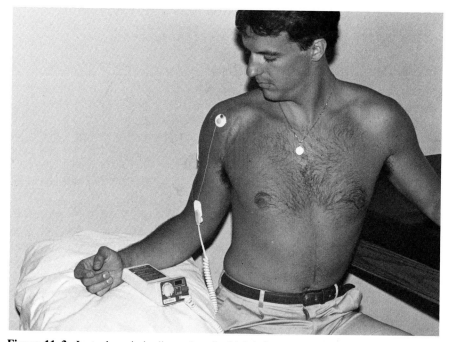

Figure 11–3 Iontophoresis is directed to the bicipital groove region. The athlete is positioned with mild external rotation and shoulder extension.

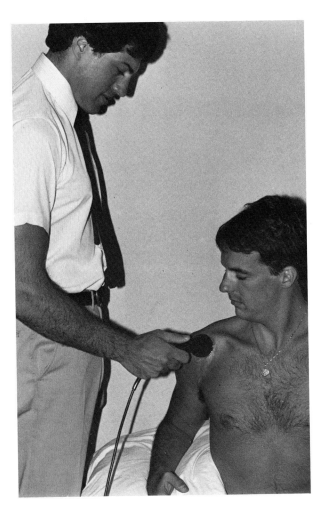

Figure 11–4 Phonophoresis to the subacromial bursa is accomplished by placing the shoulder in extension, which causes the bursa to move anteriorly.

Muscular and Capsular Stretching

Stretching the shoulder capsule and the supporting shoulder muscles should be supervised and augmented with a home program. Joint mobilization may be necessary in cases of restricted joint motion that both cause and are secondary to pain. Mobilization techniques are indicated when there is a loss of motion. This can be related to soft tissue contractures or adhesions.

The synovial joint capsule has been shown to contain sensory organs or mechanoreceptors (31) that are sensitive to range of motion, proprioception, and kinetic sense. Following injury or surgical procedures, adhesions and joint contractures may develop and interfere with these protective and adaptive end organs.

Joint mobilization and range of motion that produce pain tend to elicit reflex muscle response, which may restrict further movement of the joint. Emphasis should be placed on avoiding reflex muscle contraction that prevents or restricts desired joint movement (17). This may be accomplished by the use of manual therapy or joint mobilization techniques (2, 15, 20, 25).

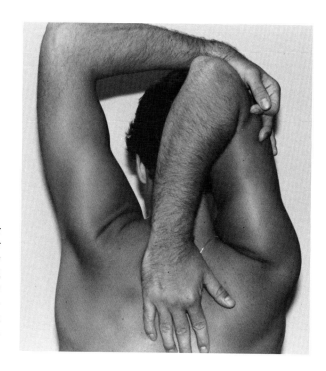

Figure 11–5 The inferior portion of the shoulder capsule is stretched by placing the arm behind and overhead with the elbow flexed. Using the uninvolved arm, this position is maintained for 60 seconds.

When the acute inflammatory stage is controlled, manual capsular stretching and pendulum exercises are begun. Pendulum exercises are an important part of the home capsular stretching program. The patient attaches a weight above the wrist and swings his arm in small circles both clockwise and counterclockwise. Emphasis is placed on relaxing the entire limb letting the weight pull the arm around. To protect the umbar spine, this exercise can be conducted with the knees bent or lying over the side of a strong table (see Figure 11–9). Home stretching, as seen in Figures 11–5 thru 11–8, may be used. During the entire rehabilitation process, functional progress should be documented.

Sawing-type motions involving the shoulder can be used as a warm-up exercise. These are started before mobilization or progressive resistive exercises are attempted in order to "warm up" the subacromial structures.

Strengthening

Low-weight, high-repetition, strengthening exercises are conducted in the side-lying and supine positions (Figures 11–10 and 11–11). Emphasis is placed on eccentric contractions in these exercises, especially for the weak external rotators. Both concentric and eccentric contractions should be used during rehabilitation (Figure 11–12). The posterior cuff muscles act to decelerate the arm in motion eccentrically during the follow-through phase of throwing (14). Eccentric loading is often overlooked in shoulder rehabilitation programs. These exercises can later be progressed to pulleys for both external and internal rotation.

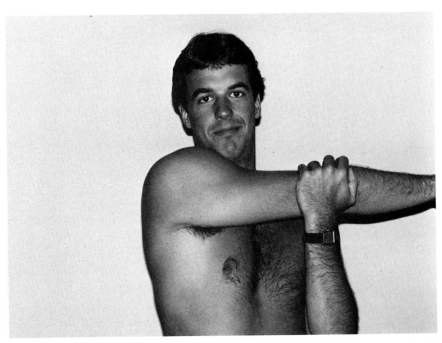

Figure 11–6 The posterior cuff and capsule are stretched here as the athlete's shoulder is placed at 90 degrees of elevation. The opposite hand is used to pull the arm into horizontal adduction with mild elbow flexion. This position is maintained for 60 seconds.

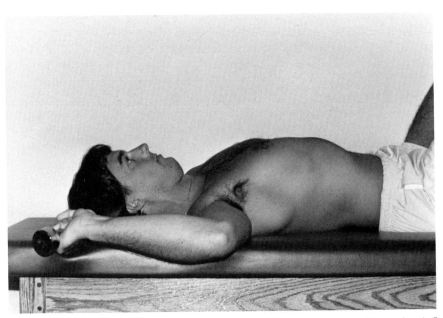

Figure 11–7 Capsular stretching can also be conducted from the supine position using 1–5 pounds of weight. Position the athlete at 90 degrees of shoulder abduction and 90 degrees of elbow flexion; let the shoulder stretch into external rotation.

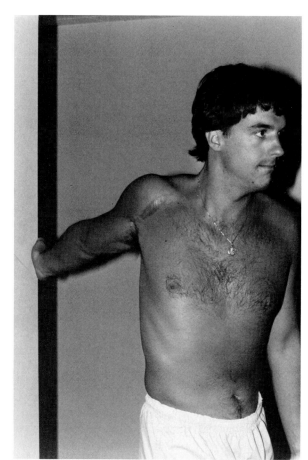

Figure 11–8 Stretching tight internal rotators can be conducted easily in a doorway. Place the athlete's palm against the doorjamb. This position places the shoulder in external rotation, extension, and horizontal abduction. The shoulders are kept parallel to the wall.

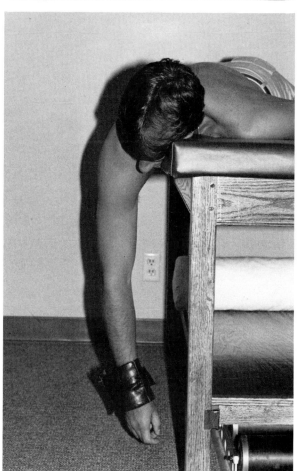

Figure 11–9 Prone pendulum exercises can be used for capsular stretching. Use weights above the wrist. This will keep forearm muscles loose.

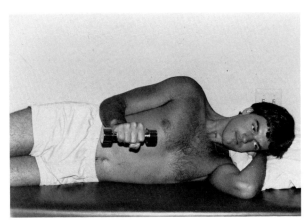

Figure 11–10 The weak external rotators can be exercised in the side-lying position. The elbow is kept on the hip as the athlete externally rotates from this neutral shoulder position. Ten to fifteen repetitions are used with light weights.

As soon as progress allows, the exercises begin to focus on the entire shoulder complex. Scapular muscles or upward rotators, such as the serratus anterior and upper trapezius, should be included (Figures 11–13 and 11–14).

Supraspinatus isolation can be used, but care should be taken when using exercises that move the greater tuberosity up into the coracoacromial arch region (12). When inflammation is present, the position of elevation and internal rotation can exacerbate impingement.

The biceps is an important muscle that helps decelerate the rapidly extending and pronated forearm during the follow-through phase of throwing (13). The biceps should also receive some attention with eccentric exercise.

Proprioceptive neuromuscular facilitation (PNF) techniques used by Knott and Voss (18) help facilitate joint receptors located in the shoulder capsule and functionally related muscles. Each pattern begins with the muscle group on stretch and ends with a maximally shortened muscle. These patterns work both the antagonist and agonist during movements. PNF techniques include scapular patterns, hold-relax motions, and slow-reversal patterns of movement. PNF can also be used

Figure 11–11 Internal rotators can be exercised from the supine position. Block out external rotation if needed because of pain or excessive soft tissue stretching.

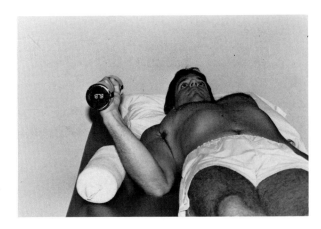

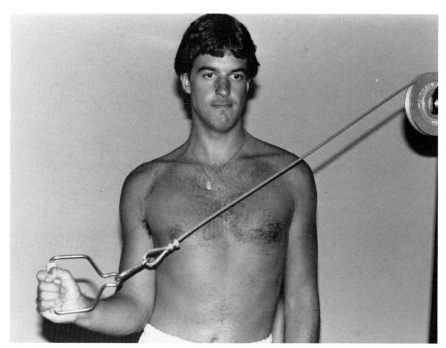

Figure 11–12 External rotators can be strengthened from a pulley-type machine. Eccentric contractions should be emphasized. The athlete can also work internal rotators on the same type of machine.

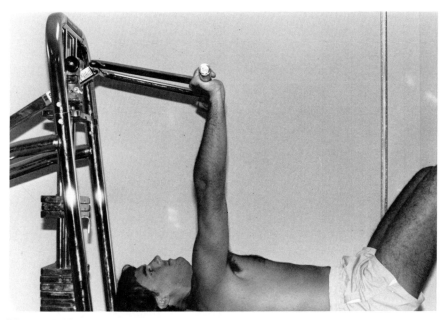

Figure 11–13 The serratus anterior, an important scapular upward rotator, is exercised off the bench press machine. The elbows are kept straight during the exercise, and the serratus anterior is used while lifting.

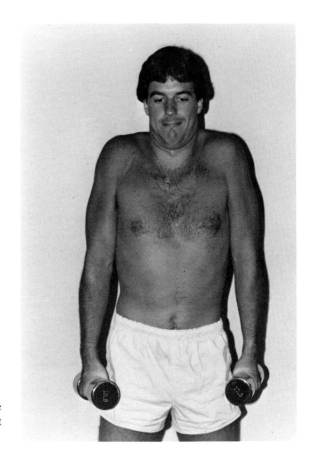

Figure 11–14 Here the athlete is using dumbells as he exercises the upper trapezius muscle, another important scapular upward rotator.

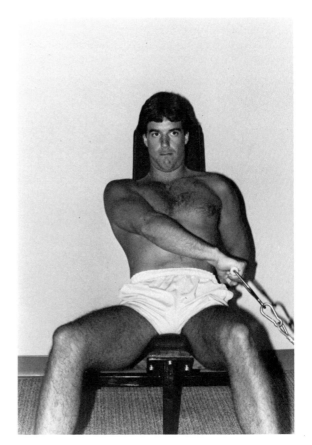

Figure 11–15 PNF patterns using light weights off a pulley-type machine are a good functional exercise. Here the athlete is shown from the starting position of the flexion-abduction-external rotation pattern. This type of exercise is used in the final stages of rehabilitation.

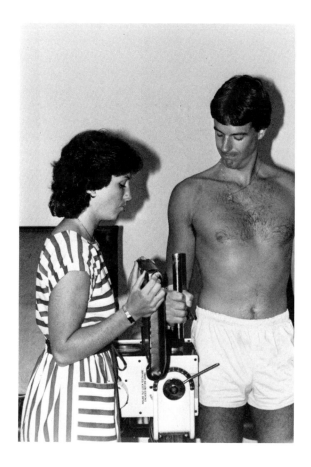

Figure 11–16 The Cybex is used to work on internal and external rotators isokinetically. A forearm strap is used to help maintain stability. Block out external rotation if necessary when treating a soft tissue repair of the anterior dislocation.

with pulleys, both in the clinic and for home programs conducted at the athlete's gym or health club (Figure 11–15).

Isokinetic exercise is an area of some controversy in rehabilitation. It can be beneficial if used selectively without overloading the injured structures. These exercises permit movement at various speeds closer to those limb velocities used during various athletic activities (Figure 11–16). Care should be taken when working the shoulder internal-external rotators from 90 degrees of shoulder abduction with elbow flexion. This position can put considerable force loads on subacromial structures and cause further dysfunction. Speed of movement for internal-external rotation can be controlled between 15–50 rpm. PNF patterns may also be used isokinetically with the Cybex during the final phases of rehabilitation if movements are pain free. Sport-specific conditioning may accomplish the same objectives but also requires supervision.

Impingement Syndrome: Postsurgical Rehabilitation

Following resection of the coracoacromial ligament or resection combined with partial acromionectomy, pendulum exercises are usually started on the second or third postoperative day. They may be started as soon as pain and patient status allow.

The patient should avoid active abduction during the first 10–14 days postoperatively especially if the deltoid muscle has been sutured. Passive shoulder flexion and active-assisted exercises are used during this early postoperative phase.

Mobilization techniques may be used to decrease muscle guarding. The patient should progress with the exercise program as tolerated and within the limits of pain. The exercise should not evoke a painful response.

Before returning to overhead activities, full, pain-free range of motion is desired. Rotator cuff strength, especially the weak external rotators, can be documented by such techniques as Cybex testing or manual testing compared to the uninvolved shoulder.

Return to Sports Activities

Film analysis has been helpful in selected athletes and may disclose factors predisposing to rotator cuff dysfunction. High-speed film analysis or shuttered videotape is ideal but not always possible.

The best surgery and rehabilitation will not help the athlete who abuses the principles of human motion (form). Elimination of poor training techniques and appropriate preventitive methods are important factors and should be discussed with the athlete's coach and trainer. For example, a pitcher may use mostly his upper body during the throwing motion. The pitcher's body may be leading or "opening up," leaving the arm behind. These motions may contribute to further shoulder dysfunction. Good pitching form enables the athlete to build momentum sequentially. Motion is transferred from the forward leg to the hips. The hips stop moving and forces are added to the torso and finally the pitching arm. The freestyle swimmer who suffers from shoulder pain and is breathing on the symptomatic side. The athlete may be alternate sides to decrease repetitive stress on the breathing-side shoulder. Additional stroke modifications may decrease force loads on the painful side. These include increasing the body roll during the recovery phase and decreasing the internal rotation during the powerful pull-through phase of swimming. Shoulder symptoms may necessitate an increase in kickboard mileage with a decrease of all strokes that cause pain. The use of training paddles can place considerable forces on the rotator cuff during the pull-through phase of the freestyle stroke and should be avoided in the swimmer with anterior shoulder pain.

Another example is the tennis player who develops shoulder pain by using the overhead stroke in a fashion that places the ball slightly behind and above the player. A change of technique that allows the player to hit the ball in front of his body may help to decrease the impingement.

The athlete's progress in sporting activity should be slow and gradual. For the baseball thrower, the "fungo drill" is an excellent example (10). This drill progresses the thrower from a long-toss position back to the pitching mound in a systematic manner.

Another consideration is the development of an impingement syndrome from the improper utilization of exercise equipment at the health club. Special attention to equipment that places the athlete internally rotated with shoulder abduction can aggravate the subacromial structures. Exercise programs can be modified to allow the athlete use of various health club equipment (3).

Rotator Cuff Repair: Postsurgical Rehabilitation

Most athletes with rotator cuff repairs are placed in the "sling position" and can begin rehabilitation during the first week postoperatively if pain and the repair permit. Pendulum exercises, mild sawing-type motions, elbow flexion-extension, and pronation-supination are performed with the shoulder adducted toward the body.

During the first month and within the limits of pain, gentle passive shoulder abduction, flexion, and internal-external rotation from the neutral position are maintained in therapy. In the second month, mild active-assisted shoulder flexion and external rotation are added to the exercise program. Isometric, external-internal rotation from the neutral position are introduced as part of the home program. Active abduction is avoided during this initial period.

A more vigorous rehabilitation program will commence during the third month, with 85–100% of full range of motion expected during this period. The exercise program initiated in the third month begins without weights, later progressing to 1- to 5-pound weights. Emphasis is still placed on maintaining mobility about the rotator cuff, and heavy strength training is avoided for at least 9–12 months.

When range of motion is reestablished, pain-free, mild ball tossing under 30 feet is started (11). Progression should continue if the athlete has no inflammatory signs or no night pain. During the fifth month the athlete may pitch a ball 60 feet, and at 6 months after surgery, a return to pitching at three-quarter speed is allowed (21). Throughout the entire rehabilitation program, general body conditioning is maintained by using the bicycle ergometer and selective lower extremity exercises.

Glenohumeral Instability

Glenohumeral instabilities are commonly symptomatic in the athletic population. The anterior and inferior glenohumeral instability patterns are the ones most commonly treated by surgery. The posterior and multidirectional instabilities are more complex and have less predictable surgical results; therefore, they are less frequently treated by surgery in the athlete. The pathomechanics of the instability are most important in the treatment program.

The rehabilitation program is based on strengthening dynamic stabilizers that oppose the direction of the instability. Care should be taken in the exercise program and sports activities to avoid further capsular stretching in the same direction as the subluxation or dislocation. Another objective of the exercise program is to improve the strength of the rotator cuff and deltoid muscles without causing mechanical irritation of the capsule and ligaments (22).

Rehabilitation can alter dynamic stability of the shoulder but does not effect the static stabilizers. If the ligaments, capsule, and bone configuration are altered significantly, instability is going to persist and be symptomatic in certain positions. These patients may respond only to surgery.

Nonoperative Management

Anterior Instability The nonoperative management of the anteroinferior instability syndrome includes dynamic strengthening of the shoulder internal rotators, specifically the subscapularis and anterior deltoid muscles. Strengthening the entire rotator cuff is also important for the athlete involved in overhead sports. During the cocking phase of throwing, when the athlete moves to what Saha (29) calls the "zero position," the rotator cuff is called upon to help glenohumeral stability (Figure 11–17).

Key points of rehabilitation include building scapular stability and general shoulder strengthening. Signs of possible impingement or inflammatory conditions need to be recognized early. Patient education is given in exercise programs conducted at the health club, especially on rotation. Avoid stretching soft tissue structures that provide static stability (24). The athlete who plays football and has anterior instability should avoid tackling with the affected arm.

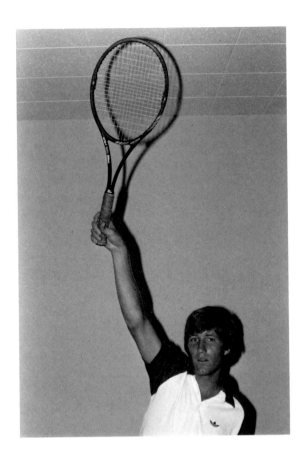

Figure 11–17 The athlete is seen here in the zero position. The head of humerus is pointing directly into the glenoid. The shoulder is abducted between 155–165 degrees overhead and 45 degrees in front of the coronal plane. All major shoulder girdle muscles are pulling the head of humerus into the glenoid to help maintain stability. When the shoulder moves out of the zero position, the small rotator cuff muscles are called upon to help maintain stability.

Posterior Instability   Recurrent posterior glenohumeral instability may occur as a result of trauma in the adducted and internally rotated position (28, 30). Posterior subluxation has been reported with the athlete in abduction with forward flexion (23). Position of injury during athletics may include linebacker recoil, crew sweep stroke, and the follow-through during overhead sports activities (23). Activities such as bench press or the arm lock in wrestling can also be compromising.

Rehabilitation of the posterior instability concentrates on strengthening the posterior cuff and posterior deltoid muscles. The exercise program should be conducted in positions of stability and away from positions of adduction with internal rotation.

Postoperative Rehabilitation

Anterior Instability   The athlete uses a sling for comfort and usually begins motion 2–6 weeks following a repair for instability. The actual length depends on the method of repair. During the protected period, limited sawing motion, pendulums, and elbow motion are encouraged. Following certain repairs for anterior instability, gentle passive shoulder flexion and abduction with internal rotation can be conducted 10 days after surgery by the therapist. Special attention to avoid excessive passive external rotation is necessary. The humeral head with a large Hill-Sachs lesion or a significant glenoid defect may require a slower approach toward rehabilitation.

Educating the patient on protection of the surgical repair is important. Certain repairs may benefit from being placed in a harness at night for at least 5–6 weeks.

Active-assisted range of motion working on shoulder flexion is usually started at 3 weeks. Mild PNF scapular patterns may supplement this phase. Isometric internal and external rotation may be introduced as early as the third or fourth week. At 5 weeks, 1- to 5-pound weights may be used within the tolerance of pain. Internal rotators should be strengthened with anterior instability and posterior rotators should be stressed with posterior instability. PNF hold-relax patterns in pain-free ranges are introduced at this time.

By the seventh to ninth postoperative week, the progression from isometrics has occurred and mild isokinetic rotator cuff exercises are started. Isokinetic exercise is done at submaximal efforts. These exercises should include limitations on the range of motion permitted. For example, in anterior instability external rotation is blocked out while only working the internal rotators. PNF slow reversals, within the range of motion, are used at this time to stimulate joint capsule receptors and muscular strength. The above protocol works with the Bristow repair. Other soft tissue repairs should progress slower.

Within five to seven months, range of motion has usually returned, with the exception of extreme external rotation. This loss of rotation has been reported to decrease performance levels during overhead sports (7).

Posterior Instability   Rehabilitation and surgical procedures for the posterior instability have many techniques and protocols. Bone blocks, glenoid osteotomies, and soft tissue structures are sometimes used for the repair.

Initial exercises are often quite limited. Avoid the position of adduction with internal rotation during early passive range of motion. Mild PNF scapular patterns can be started at 4 weeks. Isometric rotator cuff exercises may be introduced as early as the fourth week. Emphasis should be placed on the external rotators. Mild isotonic cuff exercises may commence during the seventh week. Hold-relax PNF patterns moving into flexion-abduction-external rotation will be used around 8 weeks. By 9 weeks isokinetic exercise is done at submaximal efforts with emphasis on external rotators, with limitations on internal rotation. Before the athlete is discharged, a safe gym or health club exercise program is outlined with emphasis on avoiding exercises and activities of potential risk.

Summary

Adequate rehabilitation of the shoulder will improve operative and nonoperative treatment. The athlete benefits from restoration of complete range of motion and strength. In addition, the fine tuning includes flexibility, muscular endurance and power, and general conditioning. Restoration of desired function to the greatest possible degree in the shortest time possible is the goal of most patients.

References

1. Burnet BE, Haddad RJ, Porche EB. Rotator cuff impingement syndrome in sports. Physician and Sportsmedicine 10:86–94, 1982
2. Cyriax, J. Textbook of Orthopaedic Medicine, 7th ed. Bailliere Tindall, London, 1978
3. Einhorn A. Shoulder rehabilitation: Equipment modification. J. Orthop. Sports Phys. Therapy 6(4), 1985
4. Fowler P. Swimmer problems. Am J Sports Med 7:141–142, 1979
5. Hawkins RJ, Hobeika PE. Impingement syndrome in the athletic shoulder. Clinics in Sports Medicine 2:391–405, 1983

6. Hawkins RJ, Kennedy JC. Impingement syndrome in athletes. Am J Sports Med 8:151–157, 1980

7. Hill JA, Lombardo SJ, Kerlan RK, et al. The modified Bristow-Helfet procedure for recurrent anterior shoulder subluxations and dislocations. Am J Sports Med 9:283–287, 1981

8. Hoppenfeld S. Physical Examination of the Spine and Extremities. Appleton-Century-Crofts, New York, 1976

9. Jackson DW. Chronic rotator cuff impingement in the throwing athlete. Am J Sports Med 4:231–240, 1976

10. Jobe FW. Symposium: Shoulder problems in overhead-overuse sports. Am J Sports Med 7:139–140, 1979

11. Jobe FW. Serious rotator cuff injuries. Clinics in Sports Medicine 2:407–412, 1983

12. Jobe FW, Moynes DR. Delineation of diagnostic criteria and a rehabilitation program for rotator cuff injuries. Am J Sports Med 10:336–339, 1982

13. Jobe FW, Moynes DR, Tibone JE, Perry J. An EMG analysis of the shoulder in pitching. Am J Sports Med 12:218–220, 1984

14. Jobe FW, Tibone JE, Perry J, Noynes D. An EMG analysis of the shoulder in throwing and pitching. Am J Sports Med 11:3–5, 1983

15. Kaltenborn FM. Mobilization of the Extremity Joints, 3rd ed. Olaf Norlis Bokhandel Universitetsgaten, Oslo, 1980

16. Kennedy JC, Hawkins R, Krissoff WB. Orthopaedic manifestations of swimming. Am J Sports Med 6:309–332, 1978

17. Kessler, RM, Hertling D. Management of Common Musculoskeletal Disorders, Physical Therapy Principles and Methods. Harper & Row, Philadelphia, 1983

18. Knott M, Voss D. Proprioceptive Neuromuscular Facilitation: Patterns and Techniques. Harper & Row, New York, 1968

19. Leach RE, O'Connor PO, Jones R. Acromionectomy for tendonitis of the shoulder in athletes. Physician and Sportsmedicine 7:96–107, 1977

20. Maitland GD. Peripheral Manipulation, 2nd ed. Butterworths, London, 1977

21. Moynes DR. Prevention of injury to the shoulder through exercises and therapy. Clinics in Sports Medicine 2:413–422, 1983

22. Neer CS, Foster CR. Inferior capsular shift for involuntary inferior and multidirectional instability of the shoulder. J Bone Joint Surg [Am] 62:897–908, 1980

23. Norwood LA, Terry GC. Shoulder posterior subluxation. Am J Sports Med 12:25–30, 1984

24. Pappas AM, Goss TP, Kleinman PK. Symptomatic shoulder instability due to lesions of the glenoid labrum. Am J Sports Med 11:279–288, 1983

25. Parris SV. Extremity Dysfunction and Mobilization (pre-publication edition). Institute Press, Atlanta, 1980

26. Penny HN, Welsh MB. Shoulder impingement syndrome in athletes and their surgical management. Am J Sports Med 9:11–15, 1981

27. Richardson AB. Overuse syndrome in baseball, tennis, gymnastics, and swimming. Clinics in Sports Medicine 2:379–390, 1983

28. Saha AK. Recurrent Dislocation of the Shoulder, 2nd ed. Thieme-Stratton, New York, 1981

29. Saha AK. Mechanism of shoulder movements and a plea for the recognition of "zero position" of glenohumeral joint. Clin Orthop 173:3–10, 1983

30. Samilson RL, Prieto V. Posterior dislocation of the shoulder in athletes. Clinics in Sports Medicine 2:369–378, 1983

31. Wyke BD. Articular neurology: A review. Physiotherapy 5:94–99, 1972

Acromioclavicular Injuries and Surgical Treatment

12

Thomas J. Harries
Jay S. Cox

Injuries to the acromioclavicular joint have long been recognized as a potentially difficult diagnostic and therapeutic problem. Hippocrates' writing in 400 B.C. reported on the diagnosis and conservative treatment. These injuries are usually the result of a direct blow produced by a fall on the point of the shoulder with downward force being applied to the acromion. Contact sports such as football, hockey, wrestling, and rugby have a high incidence of these injuries.

The amount of displacement of the distal clavicle following an injury to the acromioclavicular joint depends upon the extent of rupture of 1) the acromioclavicular ligament, 2) the acromioclavicular capsule, 3) the coracoclavicular ligaments, and 4) the trapezius and deltoid muscles. Horizontal stability of the clavicle depends upon the acromioclavicular ligament and vertical stability depends upon the coracoclavicular ligament.

Classification

It is important to understand the new classification of acromioclavicular injuries as recently described by Rockwood and Green (11). Previously, there had been much controversy about the treatment of type III injuries. Rockwood has attempted to clarify these complicated type III injuries by devising a new classification scheme.

The type I classification has not changed and represents a partial tear of the acromioclavicular ligament. The type II injury is a rupture of the acromioclavicular ligament with a partial tear of the coracoclavicular ligament. The distal clavicle is displaced upward in relation to the acromion, but less than the full width of the clavicle.

The type III injury is a rupture of the acromioclavicular ligament *and* a rupture of the coracoclavicular ligament with upward displacement of the distal clavicle above the level of the acromion. As mentioned previously, the amount of upward displacement of the distal clavicle depends also upon the amount of injury to the deltoid and trapezius musculature aponeurosis. A severe upward displacement in which the deltoid-trapezius aponeurosis is completely ruptured allows the distal clavicle to displace into subcutaneous tissue. The distal clavicle may also be displaced posteriorly or superiorly into the muscle fibers, trapping the clavicle and preventing reduction. Bannister et al (2) have reported that these injuries require surgical intervention in order to prevent late sequelae.

To clarify these more severe injuries, Rockwood and Green (11) have recently described the type IV injury as a type III injury with the distal clavicle displaced into or through the deltoid-trapezius aponeurosis in a "buttonhole" fashion. The clavicle cannot be reduced because it is trapped by muscle fibers. Because the distal clavicle frequently goes posteriorly into the trapezius musculature, the upward displacement on a standard anteroposterior roentgenogram may not be appreciated. Therefore, some of these injuries may be misclassified as type III injuries if only the standard view is used. In 1954 Alexander (1) described a specific x-ray view in which the posterior displacement of the distal clavicle can be appreciated. This should become a standard view for all acromioclavicular injuries.

The type V injury is a previously classified type III injury with complete rupture of the deltoid trapezius musculature. The distal clavicle is covered only by skin and subcutaneous tissue.

The type VI injury is very rare and is a disruption of the sternoclavicular joint and the acromioclavicular joint with downward displacement of the distal clavicle. It is trapped underneath the muscle aponeurosis arising from the tip of the coracoid on the coracoid itself. Both the acromioclavicular and the coracoclavicular ligaments are ruptured.

Treatment of Acute Injuries

The treatment of the type I injury is certainly not controversial and involves symptomatic treatment only. This is temporary immobilization with a sling, ice application for 24–48 hours, and anti-inflammatory agents. The patient is allowed active range-of-motion exercises immediately and usually achieves full painless range of motion by 5–7 days. At that time rehabilitation of the shoulder girdle musculature is begun, and the patient is usually fit to return to full activity in approximately 2 weeks.

The treatment of type II injuries involves two options: symptomatic treatment similar to that of type I or immobilization for 4–6 weeks in a shoulder immobilizer. The reduction must be performed manually, and the immobilizer must be applied to maintain the reduction. If the clavicle cannot be reduced manually, there is probably soft tissue intervention and the immobilizer should not be used. At the U.S. Naval Academy, we discontinue immobilization and start rehabilitation after 4 weeks. This treatment may reduce the incidence of late symptoms. Care must be taken to prevent skin maceration and ensure compliance if this treatment option is to be successful. Complications with the acromioclavicular immobilizer are 1) loss of position; 2) skin problems such as maceration, irritation, or ulceration; 3) poor patient compliance; and 4) stiffness of the shoulder, especially in older patients. The sling must be worn and the position must be maintained for a minimum of 4 weeks to assure adequate healing of the soft tissues around the acromioclavicular joint. Rehabilitation is instituted first to regain range of motion and then strength.

Bergfeld et al. (3) and Cox (6) reported that residual symptoms in type II injuries were much higher than had been previously recognized. Cox found that treatment of type II injuries with an acromioclavicular immobilizer reduced the incidence of residual symptoms when compared to symptomatic treatment. It is our opinion that residual symptoms in type II injuries are caused by the chronic subluxation of the joint, allowing abnormal stress across the joint. This may result in late degenerative arthritis. In our experience residual symptoms from type II injuries are more common than symptoms in unreduced type III complete dislocations.

If symptomatic treatment is chosen, type II injuries are treated the same way as the type I injuries. The sling is worn primarily for comfort and is discontinued when active range-of-motion exercises can be instituted. When full painless range of motion of the shoulder has been achieved, an active rehabilitation program is instituted to restore full muscle strength.

Most of the controversy involving treatment of acromioclavicular joint injuries centers around the treatment of the acute type III injuries. Treatment philosophies include "skillful neglect," which is symptomatic treatment with early motion; closed reduction with immobilization in an acromioclavicular immobilizer, as described for type II injuries; or open reduction and internal fixation. Rockwood and Green (11) have reported that over 200 variations in surgical procedures have been described for treatment of the complete dislocation of the acromioclavicular joint.

In 1974 Powers and Bach (10) conducted a survey of the chairman of the orthopaedic training programs in the United States. At that time 95% of the program chairmen preferred surgery for treatment of the type III injuries. As for method of surgery, 60% preferred temporary acromioclavicular fixation and 35%, coracoclavicular fixation. Nonoperative treatment was rarely advocated.

The management of type III injuries has changed considerably over the past few years. Glick and associates (7) did a follow-up study of 35 unreduced dislocated acromioclavicular joints in athletes treated by "skillful neglect," and they reported the majority did very well.

In 1975 Imatani et al. (8) reported on a series of patients treated prospectively either operatively or nonoperatively. Their conclusion was that a combination of minimum immobilization and early rehabilitation of the shoulder was the recommended choice of treatment.

More recently, Bjerneld and colleagues (4) reported on a 5-year follow-up study of 33 patients with complete separation that was treated conservatively with minimal immobilization and with no attempt at reduction. Thirty of 33 patients obtained satisfactory results.

Most recently, Bannister et al. (2) reported on the results of a group of patients treated prospectively with surgery of "skillful neglect" and drew the conclusion that early immobilization gave results compatible to surgery, but with lower morbidity and earlier return to full activities. They did identify a small group of patients with the type IV or V injury who did poorly with "skillful neglect" and did much better with open reduction and internal fixation.

To ascertain the current thinking on the treatment of type III acromioclavicular dislocations in the United States, one of the authors (J.S.C.) sent a questionnaire to the chairmen of orthopaedic training programs. He described a young active individual with an uncomplicated type III injury and requested their preferred method of treatment. Sixty percent of those responding stated that they would treat the uncomplicated type III acromioclavicular separations nonoperatively. Thirty-seven percent of those who elected to treat the injury nonoperatively recommended immobilization, where 63% felt that "skillful neglect" was adequate treatment. A notable exception was in the dominant extremity of a throwing athlete. Most would perform surgery to restore the anatomy. This represents a significant change from the survey conducted by Powers and Bach (10) in 1974.

These same physicians were then asked the operative method they would choose in the treatment of a type III injury. Thirty percent preferred fixation across the acromioclavicular joint and 70% preferred fixation between the coracoid and the clavicle. Of the physicians who preferred coracoclavicular fixation, 80% use either fascia, tape, wire, or suture between the coracoid and the clavicle. The remaining 20% use some type of coracoclavicular screw. This trend towards fixation between the coracoid and the clavicle also represents a change from the results obtained by Powers and Bach in a similar survey 10 years ago. At that time 60% of the physicians queried were using fixation across the acromioclavicular joint.

The group members were asked if they would excise the distal clavicle in a primary surgical repair of an acute type III injury. Only 25% recommended excision of the distal clavicle. Therefore, the trend in North America today is not to excise the distal clavicle in acute primary repair unless there has been damage to the distal clavicle. Browne et al. (5) reported in 1977 on the excision of the distal clavicle in the treatment of dislocated acromioclavicular joints. They concluded that excision of the distal clavicle did not offer significant improvement over coracoclavicular fixation alone.

In summary, there are three acceptable, recognized methods of treatment for the type III injury: 1) symptomatic or "skillful neglect," 2) closed reduction and immobilization in an acromioclavicular sling for 4–6 weeks, and 3) open reduction and internal fixation.

There is little controversy regarding the treatment of the type IV or type V injuries. In general, surgical repair is indicated. The defects in the deltoid-trapezius muscle aponeurosis should be repaired.

There are six general principles of operative surgical repair: 1) The distal clavicle is reduced and maintained by fixation between the coracoid and the clavicle or across the acromioclavicular joint. 2) The coracoclavicular ligament is repaired if possible. 3) The acromioclavicular ligament is repaired if possible. 4) The acromioclavicular joint is debrided. 5) The distal clavicle is not excised unless damaged or there are existing changes in the acromioclavicular joint. 6) The deltoid and trapezius muscle aponeurosis is repaired. This repair of the deltoid and trapezius muscle is most important in operative treatment.

For surgical repair we recommend the method described by Park et al. (9). The acromioclavicular joint is exposed by a straight incision from the acromion to the coracoid process. The clavicular origin of the deltoid is elevated with the periosteum and the acromioclavicular joint is exposed. The acromioclavicular joint is debrided if necessary. Only if there is evidence of intra-articular fracture or previous pre-existing arthritis is the distal 1.5 cm of the clavicle excised and beveled in such a way to ensure that there is no impingement with 90 degrees or greater abduction of the humerus. An attempt is made to repair the coracoclavicular ligaments if possible. If there is an avulsion from the periosteum, Bunnell-type sutures are placed in the ligament, and these sutures are subsequently fixed to the periosteum or through drill holes in the clavicle or coracoid. A velour Dacron graft is used to secure the fixation. A ¼-inch drill hole is made in a superoinferior direction through the distal clavicle at the level overlying the base of the coracoid process. The velour Dacron graft is pulled through the drill hole in the clavicle around the base of the coracoid and then secured with the clavicle fully reduced. It is important to place the knot anteriorly and/or inferiorly so that it will not be prominent sub-cutaneously over the superior portion of the clavicle.

The acromioclavicular ligament and capsule are repaired, followed by a me-ticulous repair of the deltoid and trapezius muscle aponeurosis. The skin is then closed with a subcuticular suture. Drains are not routinely used.

Postoperative immobilization consists only of a sling for comfort. Active range-of-motion exercises are instituted as soon as pain permits, usually in 3–5 days. The patient continues on these exercises until full painless range of motion is achieved; then strengthening exercises are instituted and continued until the strength equals that of the opposite uninjured shoulder musculature.

The complications of operative treatment involving pins or wires across the acromioclavicular joint include migration or breakage of the wires or pins. A larger diameter of wire can be used to prevent breakage, and a bend can be made in the end of the wire to prevent migration. There is some disruption of the articular cartilage of the acromioclavicular joint when a wire is placed across the joint.

Complications in the use of screws for fixation of the clavicle to the coracoid include loosening of the screw, breakage of the screw, and possible injury to the brachial plexus, brachial artery, or veins. When using tape or wire to fix the coracoid to the clavicle, there is the possible complication of a fracture through a drill hole or erosion through the clavicle.

Treatment of Chronic Problems

The treatment of chronic pain in symptomatic type II acromioclavicular subluxa-tions is by excision of the distal 1–2 cm of the clavicle. Care is taken to confirm that enough clavicle has been removed so that there is no impingement of the joint by taking the shoulder through a full range of motion at the time of surgery. Beveling of the distal end of the clavicle may help to avoid impingement. There is no necessity for repair or reconstruction of the coracoclavicular ligaments, but attention to repair of the deltoid and trapezius muscles is necessary in closing the wound. Care should be taken not to excise an excessive amount of distal clavicle because this may produce a floating unstable distal clavicle with weakness of the overlying musculature.

Occasionally, unreduced type III or IV injuries become symptomatic. This is generally due to muscular fatigue or weakness. Prior to any surgery an intensive physical therapy rehabilitation program is instituted. If unsuccessful, the surgical procedure of choice uses the velour Dacron graft for fixation of the clavicle to the coracoid, with the excision of the distal 1–2 cm of the clavicle. The advantages are good predictable results, early initiation of active range-of-motion exercises, and no second operation for removal of internal fixation devices.

Summary

Acromioclavicular joint dislocations can present difficult diagnostic and therapeutic problems. If handled with attention to detail, satisfactory results can be obtained. The key to treatment of type III injuries is to differentiate them from the type IV and V variations, which predictably have a poor result with conservative treatment. Surgery in the acute injury should be reserved primarily for type IV and V dislo-cations and occasionally for a type III injury of the dominant extremity in a throw-ing athlete. The deltoid and the trapezius muscle aponeurosis should be carefully repaired at the time of surgery.

References

1. Alexander OM. Radiography of the acromioclavicular articulation. Med Radiogr Photogr 30:34–39, 1954
2. Bannister GC, Wallace WA, et al. A prospective study of the treatment of acromio-clavicular dislocations. In Bateman JE, Welsh RP (eds) Surgery of the Shoulder, CV Mosby, St. Louis, 1984
3. Bergfeld JA, Andrish JT, Clancy WG. Evaluation of the acromioclavicular joint following first and second degree sprains. Am J Sports Med 6:153–159, 1978
4. Bjerneld H, Hovelius L, Thorling J. Acromioclavicular separations treated conservatively. Acta Orthop Scand 54:743–745, 1983
5. Browne J, Stanley RF, Tullos HS. Acromioclavicular joint dislocations, comparative results following operative treatment with and without primary distal clavisectomy. Am J Sports Med 5:258–263, 1977
6. Cox JS. The fate of the acromioclavicular joint in athletic injuries. Am J Sports Med 9:50–53, 1981
7. Glick JM, Milburn LJ, Haggerty JF, Nishimoto D. Dislocated acromioclavicular joint: Follow-up study of 35 unreduced acromioclavicular dislocations. Am J Sports Med 5:264–270, 1977
8. Imatani RJ, Hanlon JJ, Cady GW. Acute complete acromioclavicular separations. J Bone Joint Surg [Am] 57:328–331, 1975
9. Park JP, Arnold JA, Coker TP, et al. Treatment of acromioclavicular separations. Am J Sports Med 8:251–256, 1980
10. Powers JA, Bach PJ. Acromioclavicular separation closed or open treatment. Clin Orthop 104:213–223, 1974
11. Rockwood CA, Green OP. Fractures in Adults, 2nd ed, vol 1, p 860. JB Lippincott, Philadelphia, 1984

Surgical Treatment of Anterior Dislocation of the Shoulder

13

James M. Colville
Douglas W. Jackson

Incidence

Anterior instability of the glenohumeral joint is a common cause of shoulder disability in the athletically active population. The overall incidence of traumatic anterior dislocation of the shoulder has been reported between 10.3 and 11.7 per 100,000 individuals (20, 42). The incidence is roughly two to three times greater in males than females. The athletically inclined population is at a significantly higher risk for this injury than the general population, accounting for between 25% and 47% of such injuries in published series. Hovelius (19) reported an incidence of traumatic dislocations of 8% in a population of Swedish ice hockey players over the course of a single season, and Jobe and Jobe (22) have stated that anterior dislocation is the second most common shoulder problem in an athletic population.

Pathology

The shoulder has the widest useful range of motion of any joint and has correspondingly few bony constraints. The glenoid cavity itself is small and shallow, causing Rockwood (37) to compare the bony stability of the shoulder to "nailing a saucer on a wall, and asking it to hold a basketball." The joint relies on soft tissue capsular, ligamentous, and muscular constraints for stability. When the humeral head is levered forward out of the glenoid fossa, damage may occur to these constraints. The static stabilizers of the anterior shoulder consist of the glenoid

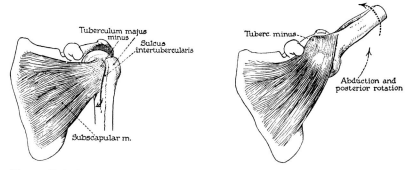

Figure 13-1 Subscapularis tendon slipping dorsally in external rotation and abduction thus "uncovering" the humeral head which is now only restrained by capsular element. [Reproduced with permission from Magnuson P, Stack J. JAMA 123:889–892, 1943]

labrum and the capsule, including the superior, middle, and inferior glenohumeral ligaments. Dynamic stabilization anteriorly is provided by the subscapularis muscle-tendon unit and to some extent, perhaps, the short head of the biceps and the anterior deltoid. As the humerus is put into abduction and external rotation, the subscapularis rotates superiorly, thus "uncovering" the humeral head (Figure 13–1). This leaves only the glenoid labrum, capsule, and ligaments restraining the head, "the position of risk" for dislocation.

As the humerus moves forward during a dislocation, the glenoid labrum may be avulsed from its attachment (sometimes taking a bit of the glenoid rim) and the head slides between the glenoid and the labrum, stripping periosteum off the anterior capsule (Figure 13–2). This is the classic Bankart lesion. Often after reduction the periosteum and capsule do not reattach to the scapular neck, instead becoming adherent to the overlying subscapularis tendon. Thus a persistent weak area is created, which may predispose to recurrence.

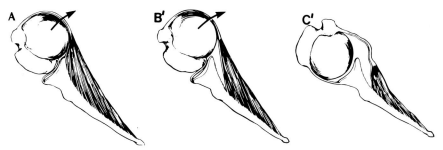

Figure 13-2 As the humeral head moves forward (**A**) the glenoid labrum is avulsed from the bone, and the periosteum under the subscapularis strips off the scapular neck (**B**). After relocation, often the periosteum does not reattach to the scapular creating the classic Bankart lesion (**C**). [Reproduced with permission from Rockwood CA. In: Rockwood CA, Green DP (eds). JB Lippincott, Philadelphia, 1984]

Table 13–1 Incidence of Hill-Sachs Lesions in Published Series

Authors	No. of Cases	Notch Present	%
Flower (12)	41	41	100
Joessel (23)			report
Broca (5)			report
Perthes (35)	2	2	100
Schultze (40)	24	5	20
Pilz (36)	21	15	71
Hermodsson (15)	40	33	82
Hill-Sachs (16)	15	11	74
Bost (3)	10	10	100
Eyre Brook (11)	17		64
Adams (1)	68	56	82
Palmer (34)	60	60	100
Townley (44)	58		"usual"
Brar (4)	65	41	67
Rowe (38)	63		57
Du Toit (10)	147		33
Moseley (32)			"usual"
MacDonald (25)	58	50	
De Anguim (6)	200	200	100
De Palma (9)			35–50

Alternatively, if the glenoid labrum does not detach and the capsular ligaments are merely stretched, the same loss of stability may be produced, but rather than the Bankart lesion, an attenuated, baggy capsule with a stretched or traumatized subscapularis tendon is produced. This lesion has been described as "the" essential lesion by Osmond-Clarke (33).

Magnuson and Stack (26) observed that as the humerus is put into the position of risk, the subscapularis tendon tends to sublux superiorly, and they felt that recurrences were caused by pathology within the muscle-tendon unit which allowed an abnormal degree of motion, thus uncovering the humeral head more than normal. They felt that a relative muscle imbalance was thereby created, predisposing to recurrent dislocation.

The presence of a posterior humeral head defect, the Hill-Sachs lesion, was described by Flower (12) in 1861. This lesion is present to a greater or lesser degree in anywhere from 25% to 100% of recurrently dislocating shoulders (see Table 13–1). The lesion is thought to be a compression fracture caused by the traumatic passage of the soft posterior humeral head over the sharp anterior lip of the glenoid (Figure 13–3). Once present, this lesion will tend to destabilize the humerus in the glenoid fossa, with the head in external rotation.

Ever since Bankart (2) described his "essential lesion," there has been a controversy as to where the critical pathology lies that predisposes to recurrent dislocation. In any given case, any or all of these lesions may be present, as well as congenital abnormalities in the angle and shape of the glenoid and humeral head, fractures of the humeral head or glenoid, and abnormalities of the rotator cuff. Conversely, there does not appear to be any single lesion that is present in all cases. The surgeon should have in his armanentarium a variety of techniques that will allow him to individualize treatment based on the pathology present.

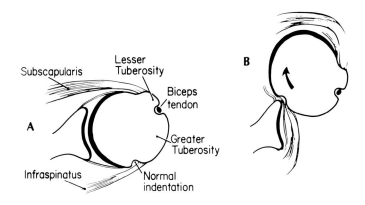

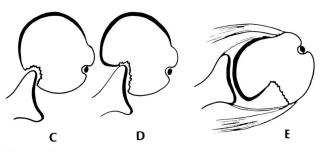

Figure 13-3 A horizontal section through the glenohumeral joint shows the formation of a posterolateral humeral head defect. **(A)** Normal anatomical relationships. **(B)** Anterior dislocation without a compression fracture defect. **(C)** A small posterolateral defect. **(D)** A large compression fracture defect. **(E)** Following reduction, the defect is quite evident and has deformed the normal articular surface of the humeral head. [Reproduced with permission from Rockwood CA. In: Rockwood CA, Green DP (eds). JB Lippincott, Philadelphia, 1984]

Natural History

Once a traumatic dislocation requiring reduction has occurred, the question arises for the patient and the treating surgeon as to when, if ever, surgical repair is indicated. Watson-Jones (45), who was perhaps the strongest proponent of conservative care, maintained that he had never seen a redislocation in a shoulder that had had a prompt reduction and was then treated with at least 3 weeks of immobilization in adduction and internal rotation. This contention has been disputed and not duplicated by more recent authors, who have found that recurrent dislocation may occur despite so-called "adequate" treatment. Rowe (38) and others (21, 28) have found no correlation between the period of immobilization and the incidence of recurrence. Rowe noted that those shoulders that had dislocated with relatively minor trauma had a higher rate of redislocation. Moseley (31) noted that redislocation is as much as six times more common in men than women. Several authors (29, 38, 41) have shown a positive correlation between the age at initial dislocation and the rate of recurrence: those patients who suffer their initial dislocation under the age of 20 have a redislocation rate as high as 92%, whereas those in the 20- to 40-year range show roughly a 60% dislocation rate, and those over 40, less than 15%. The majority of those who do redislocate will do so within 2 years; thereafter the incidence drops sharply. There has been some dispute in the literature as to whether these series of patients reflect selected population of persons more prone to dislocate. Simonet and Cofield (41) were able to follow a large, relatively stable unit of the general population for a period of 10 years, noting all cases of dislocation and redislocation. Of the persons who dislocated initially in that study, only 33% redislocated within 10 years. However, the rate of recurrence was 66% in those under 20 years of age, and 40% in those under 40. Although these rates are somewhat lower than those reported earlier, it is significant that 82% of the young athletes experienced redislocation, while only 30% of the nonathletes did. One may therefore conclude from the available literature that a male athlete under the age of 20 has an exceptionally high probability of recurrent dislocation.

Surgical Treatment

There have been a number of operations described to treat recurrent dislocations of the shoulder, with one of the earliest being by Hippocrates circa 400 B.C. Hippocrates used a red-hot iron to cauterize the anterior and inferior shoulder capsule and then bound the arm tightly to the side for an extended period to encourage scar formation. Recent authors have suggested more modern techniques, substituting "cold steel" for "hot iron" (37).

Five surgical procedures have been selected for discussion because of their widespread use in the athletic population to treat recurrent anterior dislocation. Tendon substitution procedures, such as the Nicola, and the true bone-block transfers, such as the Eden-Hybinette repair, have not been included, primarily because of the limited reported experience in the athletic population.

Bankart Procedure

Although Perthes was probably the first to perform this repair, in 1939 Bankart (2) published a now classic paper that detailed his concept of capsular avulsion producing a weak area anteriorly, leading to recurrent dislocations. He then described the surgical repair of the ruptured capsule to prevent further episodes. His procedure was further modified by Rowe et al. (39), and essentially it is this technique that is used in the athletic population.

General endotracheal anesthesia is induced, with the patient in the supine (Rowe does not use semisitting) position. A folded towel or blanket is placed under the scapula to permit posterior displacement of the humeral head. A straight incision is used from the palpable tip of the coracoid process to the anterior axilla. A shorter incision can be used for females. The subcutaneous tissue is divided and the deltopectoral interval is identified and developed to expose the cephalic vein. Rowe advocates ligation of the vein proximally and distally to avoid oozing. Others, including the authors, preserve the cephalic vein and retract it medially with a few fibers of the deltoid. The subscapularis muscle and tendon with their overlying fascia are then exposed, with the conjoint tendon lying at the medial aspect of the wound (Figure 13–4).

Hoppenfeld and DeBoer (18) have described two variations in the exposure of the anterior shoulder mechanism. In the first, a 10- to 15-cm straight incision is made, beginning over the coracoid process and following the deltopectoral groove distally and laterally. This is the so-called "sabre incision," and again, the deltopectoral interval is developed as before. The second variation calls for the patient's arm to be abducted 90 degrees and externally rotated. An incision of 8–10 cm is made, beginning at the midpoint of the anterior axillary fold and extending posteriorly into the axilla. Blunt dissection is used to mobilize the subcutaneous tissue anteriorly, and the skin flaps are then retracted to give exposure to the

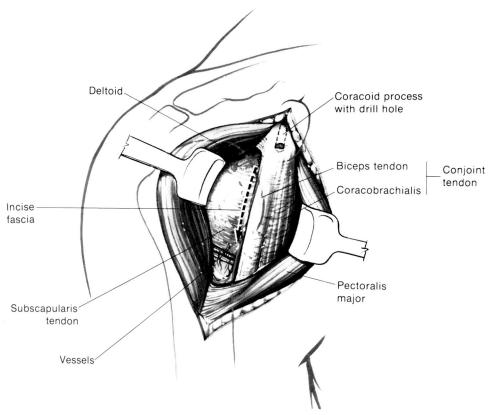

Figure 13-4 The anterior shoulder mechanism exposed. Note that the coracoid process has been drilled prior to osteotomy to facilitate reattachment. [Reproduced with permission from Hoppenfeld S, DeBoer P. Surgical Exposures in Orthopaedics: The Anatomic Approach. JB Lippincott, Philadelphia, 1984]

deltopectoral interval. The axillary incision is said to be more cosmetically appealing. We have found it technically compromising in the athletic population, particularly in the patient with a muscular shoulder.

Once exposure of the anterior shoulder mechanism is established, Rowe osteotomizes the coracoid between the conjoint tendon and the pectoralis minor insertion. It is then allowed to retract medially. The tip can be predrilled with a 2.0-mm drill and tapped prior to the osteotomy to facilitate reattachment if desired, although Rowe does not advocate this. Many shoulder surgeons do not take down the coracoid or conjoint tendon. If properly done and reattached, it does not appear to be associated with disability. It does make the exposure easier, particularly when only one assistant is used.

The arm is then turned into external rotation, bringing the subscapularis muscle and tendon into maximal exposure. The inferior border is marked by a plexus of vessels, which may be ligated or cauterized. Beginning at the inferior border of the subscapularis, the muscle and tendon are separated off the capsule of the shoulder anteriorly (Figure 13–5). This requires sharp dissection, taking care not to enter the capsule below. The tendon is detached from its insertion on the lesser tuberosity, tagged for reattachment, and retracted medially, exposing the capsule.

With the arm externally rotated, a vertical incision is made through the capsule, 0.5 cm from the glenoid rim (Figure 13–6). A humeral head retractor is then

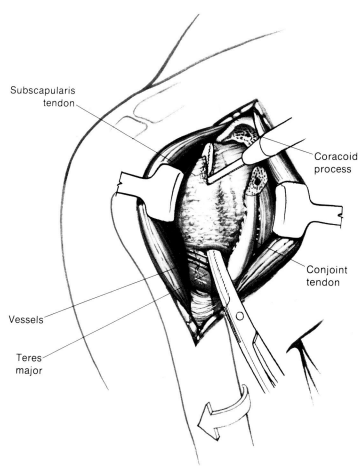

Subscapularis
tendon

Coracoid
process

Conjoint
tendon

Vessels

Teres
major

Figure 13-5 The subscapularis tendon is separated off the capsule of the shoulder anteriorly. A leash of vessels at the caudal end of the wound marks the inferior border of the tendon. It is detached from its insertion on the lesser tuberosity, dissected free, and retracted medially. [Reproduced with permission from Hoppenfeld S, DeBoer P. Surgical Exposures in Orthopaedics: The Anatomic Approach. JB Lippincott, Philadelphia, 1984]

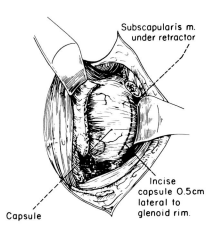

Shoulder in complete
external rotation

Subscapularis m.
under retractor

Incise
capsule 0.5cm
lateral to
glenoid rim.

Capsule

Figure 13-6 With the arm externally rotated, a vertical incision is made through the capsule 0.5 cm from the glenoid rim. [Reproduced with permission from Rowe CR. J Bone Joint Surg [Am] 38:957–977, 1956]

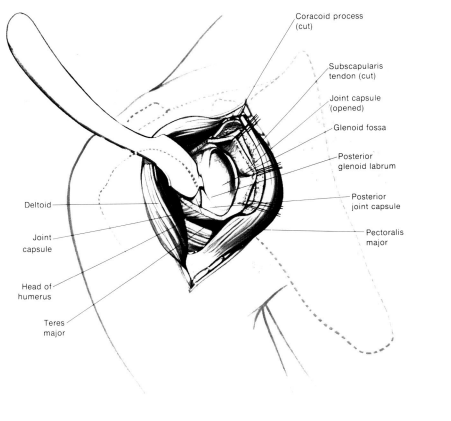

Coracoid process
(cut)

Subscapularis
tendon (cut)

Joint capsule
(opened)

Glenoid fossa

Posterior
glenoid labrum

Posterior
joint capsule

Pectoralis
major

Deltoid

Joint
capsule

Head of
humerus

Teres
major

Figure 13-7 A bankart skid is used to displace the humeral head posteriorly, exposing the glenoid cavity. [Reproduced with permission from Hoppenfeld S, DeBoer P. Surgical Exposures in Orthopaedics: The Anatomic Approach. JB Lippincott, Philadelphia, 1984]

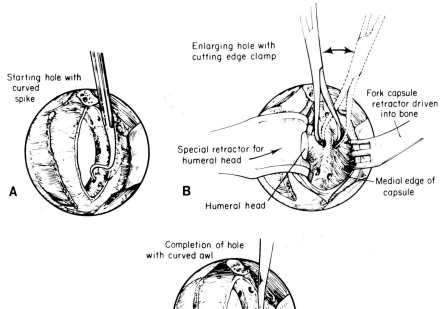

Starting hole with
curved spike

Enlarging hole with
cutting edge clamp

Fork capsule
retractor driven
into bone

Special retractor for
humeral head

Medial edge of
capsule

Humeral head

A

B

Completion of hole
with curved awl

C

Figure 13-8 Holes are made in the anterior rim in three places, as shown. **(A)** Holes are started with a curved spike, **(B)** enlarged using a cutting clamp, **(C)** completed using a curved awl. [Reproduced with permission from Rowe CR. J Bone Joint Surg [Am] 38:957–977, 1956]

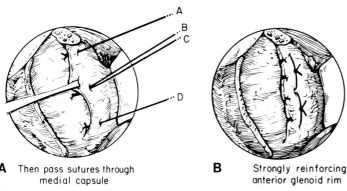

A Then pass sutures through medial capsule

B Strongly reinforcing anterior glenoid rim

Figure 13-9 One end of the superior and inferior sutures and both strands of the middle suture are left long and brought through the medial capsular flap as shown (**A**). They are then tied (**B**) giving a "pants and vest" closure to reinforce the repair. [Reproduced with permission from Rowe CR. J Bone Joint Surg [Am] 38:957–977, 1956]

placed into the joint (Figure 13–7) and used to displace the head laterally and posteriorly, thus exposing the glenoid.

If a Bankart lesion is present, three small holes are then made in the anterior rim with a dental drill or a small awl at 1, 3, and 5 o'clock on right shoulders, and at 11, 9, and 7 o'clock on left shoulders (Figure 13–8). These serve as reattachment points for the capsule. Three nonabsorbable sutures are used to fasten the capsule back to the rim. One end of the superior and inferior sutures is left long, as are both ends of the middle suture. These long ends are then brought anteriorly through the still free medial capsular flap, and tied as shown (Figure 13–9), giving a "pants and vest" reenforcement of the anterior capsular rim.

If no Bankart lesion is found, a capsular imbrication is performed.

The subscapularis tendon is then reattached to its previous position. At this point, it should be possible to passively externally rotate the arm 25 to 30 degrees with ease. The coracoid process is reattached with nonabsorbable sutures or with a screw.

Postoperative management consists of a sling used for 2 or 3 days only; then exercises are begun. Pendulum exercises are started first, and Rowe instructs patients to position the hands anterior to the coronal plane of the body for 6 weeks. He further recommends a towel under the elbow in the recumbent position for the first week to maintain slight forward flexion. By 3 months swimming, rowing, and light sports are permitted and by 6 months a complete recovery of power and range of motion is expected.

Putti-Platt Procedure

According to Osmond-Clarke (33), the operation bearing their names was originated independently in the early 1920s by Platt in England and Putti in Italy. They did not recognize the Bankart lesion as the sole source of recurrent dislocation and felt that the stretching of the anterior structures, especially the capsule and ligaments, resulted in a loss of anterior restraint. Their solution was a capsular imbrication and an imbrication of the subscapularis tendon in order to reenforce the repair. Since neither Putti or Platt published the details of their technique, the procedure given is that described by Osmond-Clarke (33).

The anterior aspect of the shoulder is exposed by any of the previously described approaches. Osmond-Clarke advocates detachment of the medial one-third of the deltoid to facilitate exposure, but few other authors have found this

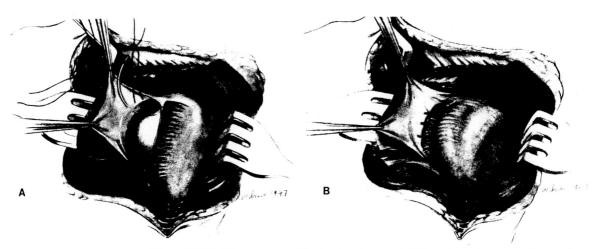

Figure 13-10 After exposure of the joint, sutures are laid from the periosteum at the anterior rim of the glenoid **(A)** and passed through the lateral capsular flap. These are then tied down **(B)** completing the first part of the capsular imbrication. Subsequently, the medial capsular flap is tacked down over the now-closed capsule completing the repair. [Reproduced with permission from Watson-Jones R. Fractures and Joint Injuries, 4th ed. Williams & Wilkins, Baltimore, 1957]

necessary. Rather than osteotomize the coracoid, Osmond-Clarke severed the conjoint tendon, taking care not to damage the musculocutaneous nerve. The tendon is then gently retracted downward and medially. Severing of the conjoint tendon is not done by the authors when using this procedure.

The subscapularis tendon is bluntly dissected free of the anterior capsule as described previously (Figure 13–5), with the arm in external rotation. The tendon is divided sharply 2.5 cm medial to its insertion. The freed tendon is retracted medially, and if the capsule is not open, it is then incised 0.5–1 cm from its anterior glenoid attachment. The joint is then examined, and any loose bodies or debris are removed. The distal stump of the subscapularis tendon and lateral edge of the capsule are then sutured down to the periosteum of the anterior edge of the glenoid (Figure 13–10). If the periosteum has been torn free of the anterior neck of the scapula, the bone should be roughened, and the lateral capsule should be sutured to the deep surface of the stripped periosteum. Four sutures are laid in and then tied while the limb is in the internal rotation. The medial edge of the capsule is then sutured down over the lateral flap, giving a pants and vest closure. As a further reenforcement, the free subscapularis muscle-tendon unit is drawn over the repaired capsule and sutured to the fascia of the bicipital groove (not into the tendon within it) or to the rotator cuff tendinous insertion on the greater tuberosity. It should be possible to externally rotate the arm to neutral at the conclusion. The conjoint tendon is then repaired, and if the deltoid has been detached, it too is replaced, and the wound is closed. The West Point modification of the Putti-Platt procedure involves tightening of the inferior glenohumeral ligament. This is accomplished by dissecting out the anteroinferior capsule and suturing it superiorly and laterally over the lateral capsule and into the lateral stump of the subscapularis tendon.

The limb is immobilized across the chest for 3–4 weeks, and then pendulum exercises are begun. No external rotation exercises are permitted before 6 weeks, after which a general program of active exercises is begun to increase strength and range of motion. Full recovery is expected within 6 months, but there will be a mild to moderate permanent loss in external rotation.

Magnuson-Stack Procedure

In 1943 Magnuson and Stack (26) published the details of a procedure to prevent recurrent anterior dislocation of the shoulder by transplantation of the subscapularis tendon. They and other authors (8, 43) felt that the primary anatomical defect predisposing to recurrence was excessive laxity of this tendon and that tightening and, to some extent, realignment of the tendon will prevent its proximal migration and resultant uncovering of the humeral head. The simplicity of the procedure together with a low rate of failure have combined to make it one of the most popular repairs in current use.

The anterior aspect of the shoulder is exposed by a deltopectoral incision. The deltopectoral interval is developed as before, exposing the subscapularis tendon insertion on the anterior aspect of the humeral head and lesser tuberosity. By externally rotating the shoulder, the tendon is brought into maximum view. By blunt and sharp dissection, a smooth retractor is inserted deep to the tendon, approximately 2.5 cm medial to its insertion (Figure 13–11). Two parallel incisions are made along the upper and lower borders of the tendon, and an osteotome is inserted into the tendon's lateral attachment, just medial to the bicipital groove, freeing the entire distal end of the tendon with a small wedge of bone. Care is taken not to injure any of the structures within the groove. The tendon is then lifted medially, together with the underlying capsule, and the joint is inspected. Loose bodies and labral remnants are removed. The arm is then internally rotated, and after the capsule is separated off, the tendon is drawn across the bicipital groove. A site of attachment lateral to the bicipital groove is selected and an osteotome is used to cut a groove in this area. Then the cut end of the subscapularis tendon with its bone fragment is wedged into the groove. The tendon is then sutured into place, using heavy interrupted sutures and taking care to anchor the superior, lateral, and inferior borders. DePalma and Silberstein (7) move the insertion distally on the humerus, as well as laterally, to prevent the humeral head from uncovering in abduction and external rotation. Gianestras (13) has described a modification in which the tendon without bone is anchored into a prepared groove with nonabsorbable sutures. The tendon can also be fixed with a staple or with AO cortical bone screw and tissue washer.

Postoperative treatment consists of a Velpeau dressing worn 3–4 weeks, after which pendulum exercises are begun. At 6 weeks the sling is discarded and full

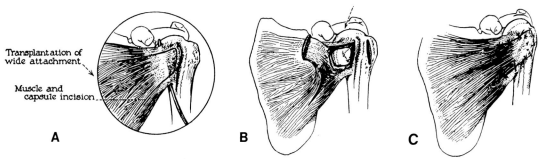

Figure 13-11 A smooth retractor is placed beneath the subscapularis tendon, 2.5 cm medial to its insertion and two parallel incisions are made along the superior and inferior borders of the tendon (**A**). Laterally, an osteotome is used to free the lateral insertion of the tendon with a small piece of bone, and connect the superior and inferior incisions (**B**). Completed repair-cut end of subscapularis tendon advanced laterally and sutured into greater tuberosity across the bicipital groove (**C**). [Reproduced with permission from Magnuson P, Stack J. JAMA 123:889–892, 1943]

active exercises are begun. A mild permanent loss of external rotation is observed, which has been measured at approximately 10 degrees on the average but has been noted to be up to 25 degrees when tested functionally with the Cybex system (30).

Bristow-Helfet Procedure

This procedure was first described in 1958 by Arthur Helfet (14), who attributed it to his late chief, W. R. Bristow. It has come into widespread use in the athletic population. The technique adds anterior bone stock to the glenoid rim; provides a musculotendinous sling, reenforcing the inferior glenohumeral ligament with the short head of biceps (especially in the abducted and externally rotated position); and finally, prevents superior subluxation of the subscapularis tendon by a tenodesis effect. The technique as modified by May (27) is the most widely used.

The patient is placed in the semisitting position, with the shoulder raised by a small sandbag or towel beneath the scapula. A sabre incision is made, as described previously, directly over the coracoid process, and the deltopectoral interval is developed. The conjoint tendon is exposed and adventitious tissue is removed from around its insertion into the tip of the coracoid (1.3 cm). The coracoid is then

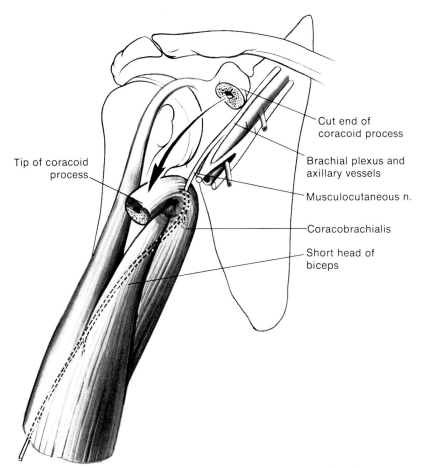

Cut end of coracoid process

Tip of coracoid process

Brachial plexus and axillary vessels

Musculocutaneous n.

Coracobrachialis

Short head of biceps

Figure 13-12 Coracoid process osteotomized and biceps retracted inferiorly. Note position of musculocutaneous nerve entering 3 cm to 4 cm distal to coracoid. [Reproduced with permission from Hoppenfeld S, DeBoer P. Surgical Exposures in Orthopaedics: The Anatomic Approach. JB Lippincott, Philadelphia, 1984]

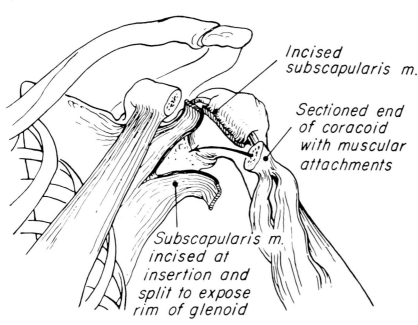

Incised
subscapularis m.

Sectioned end
of coracoid
with muscular
attachments

Subscapularis m.
incised at
insertion and
split to expose
rim of glenoid

Figure 13-13 Tendon and capsule are incised transversely, and the subscapularis tendon split longitudinally exposing the neck of the scapular and glenoid rim. [Reproduced with permission from May VR. J Bone Joint Surg [Am] 52:1010–1016, 1970]

osteotomized between the conjoint tendon and the pectoralis minor insertion. The conjoint tendon is then carefully freed distally for 3–4 cm. The musculocutaneous nerve enters the coracobrachialis muscle belly approximately 6 cm distally to the coracoid, and caution must be exercised not to injure it (Figure 13–12). The muscle and tendon of the subscapularis are exposed lying across the anterior capsule of the shoulder. The tendon and joint capsule are incised transversely just medial to the insertion on the lesser tuberosity. The joint is then exposed and inspected. The subscapularis tendon is then split longitudinally approximately 5 cm, and the underlying periosteum on the neck of the scapula is raised and the bone is freshened (Figure 13–13). A 2.8-mm hole is then drilled into the anterior neck just medial to the glenoid rim, where the coracoid is to be attached. A 1.9-cm cortical bone screw is placed through the predrilled coracoid tip, and the conjoint tendon is then passed over the inferior slip of the subscapularis tendon and anchored to the scapular neck. The transected ends of both the superior and inferior slips of the subscapularis tendon are then plicated back to their origins, using chromic suture, and the wound is closed (Figure 13–14).

A Velpeau dressing is used to maintain the shoulder in adduction and internal rotation for 4 weeks, then gentle active and passive range-of-motion exercises are begun. Although this procedure was originally touted as one that would not limit external rotation, May (27) reported up to a 15-degree loss in his patients, while Hill et al. (17) found a mean loss of 12-degrees.

Arthroscopic Staple Capsulorrhaphy

Arthroscopic surgery about the shoulder is a comparatively recent development, and the surgeon should be thoroughly familiar with the techniques of arthroscopy before attempting this repair. Arthroscopic repair of the anterior shoulder capsule has not been in wide use for enough time to permit adequate long-term

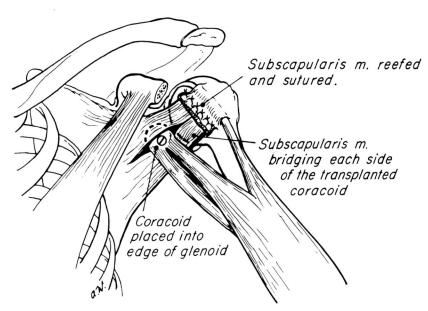

Subscapularis m. reefed and sutured.

Subscapularis m. bridging each side of the transplanted coracoid

Coracoid placed into edge of glenoid

Figure 13-14 Completed repair is shown: the conjoint tendon with coracoid tip fastened at glenoid rim over split subscapularis tendon. The subscapularis tendon is reattached to its origin at the humerous with a short plication. [Reproduced with permission from May VR. J Bone Joint Surg [Am] 52:1010–1016, 1970]

evaluation of results. However, because it offers potential advantages to athletes, such as minimal invasion, minimal alteration of normal shoulder mechanics, short hospitalization or outpatient surgery, and quick rehabilitation, it is included in this discussion. The technique and largest experience to date are attributable to Lanny Johnson (24). Several variations on types of repairs are being evaluated in other institutions.

The patient is placed in the standard position for shoulder arthroscopy, i.e., the lateral decubitus position. The arm can either be held by an assistant or can be abducted from 30–60 degrees and slightly flexed in Bucks traction, using a pulley and 10 pounds of weight. The shoulder and arm are then prepped and draped, giving access to the anterior, superior, and posterior aspects of the joint. An 18-gauge spinal needle is inserted into the joint from a point 2 cm inferior and 2 cm medial to the most lateroposterior tip of the acromion (soft spot). The joint is distended with saline and checked for reflux to be sure of proper placement, and the needle is withdrawn after noting its course. Then a 30-degree arthroscope is inserted through a stab wound in the same position, aiming for the coracoid process. Position in the joint is confirmed by direct visualization.

An 18-gauge spinal needle is then introduced into the joint under direct vision, entering through the sulcus between the clavicle and the spine of the scapula, just medial to the acromion. Its course is noted, and an inflow cannula is introduced along the same path. Thus adequate inflow and outflow (through the scope) are achieved without restricting access to the anterior joint. A complete arthroscopic examination of the joint includes noting if a Hill-Sachs lesion is present and the status of the labrum and glenohumeral ligaments (Figure 13–15).

An entry portal is selected on the anterosuperior capsular wall. This is usually just below and anterior to the biceps tendon, between the superior and middle glenohumeral ligaments. The scope is then advanced directly against this point, and while the cannula is held tightly against the anterior wall, the eyepiece is withdrawn. A Wissinger rod is inserted down the cannula and bluntly forced out the anterior shoulder so that the point rests subcutaneously, tenting the skin. The skin is incised sharply over the tip, and the rod is brought through. Then the cannula for the chondral abraider is passed retrograde back over the rod and into the joint. The rod is withdrawn, and the eyepiece is replaced in the arthroscope cannula while the chondral abraider is placed down the anterior cannula. The abraider is used under direct vision to clean and roughen the anterior rim and neck of the glenoid. This preparation will aid in the soft tissue-to-bone healing as part of the capsular repair. The staple-driver cannula is then positioned in the midportion of the anterior capsule under direct vision. Once a satisfactory position is achieved, the blunt obturator of the staple-driver cannula is withdrawn, and the staple and driver assembly is inserted into the joint. One arm of the staple is then inserted through the capsular tissue of the detached or stretched middle and/or inferior glenohumeral ligament and capsule (Figure 13–16). The staple is positioned to tighten and reapproximate these structures. It is driven into the roughened anterior neck, under direct vision. If it is not possible to tighten these structures, a portion of the subscapularis tendon can be stapled instead. The arm should be adducted and internally rotated just prior to driving in the staple. The instruments are withdrawn, fluid expressed, and the minor wounds are closed. Checking the roentgenographic position of the staple is recommended in the operating room.

A Velpeau dressing is used for 3–4 weeks to permit reattachment of the imbricated capsule, and then gentle pendulum exercises are begun. At 6 weeks unrestricted exercises to restore range of motion and power are allowed.

New instruments and techniques are being developed in several centers for variations of this type of arthroscopic repair. It appears very promising in selected cases, and its use will be further delineated in the next few years.

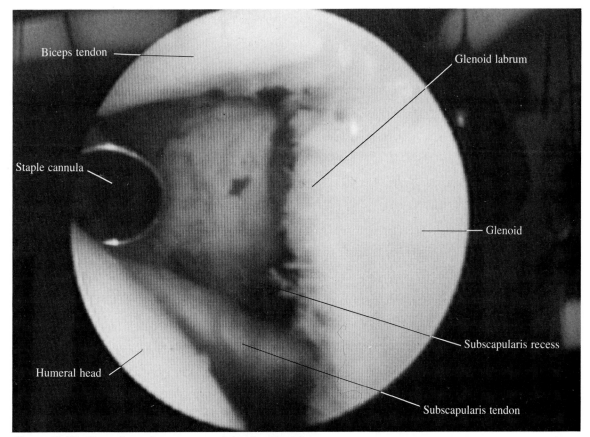

Figure 13-15 View of anterior structures of the shoulder joint.

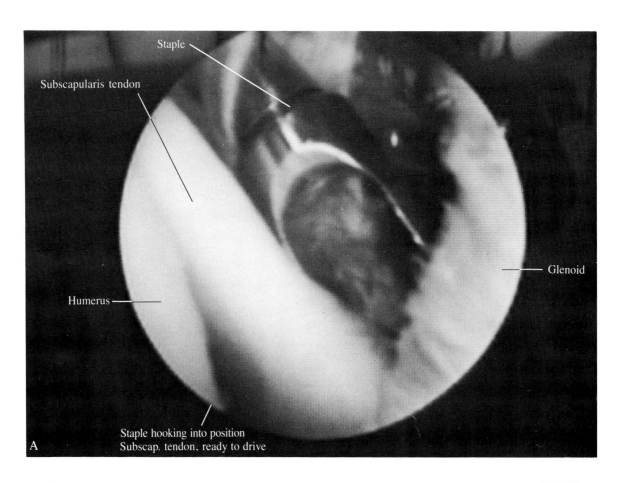

A Staple hooking into position
Subscap. tendon, ready to drive

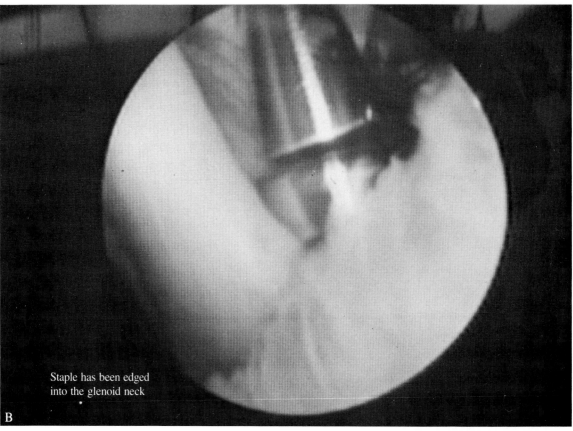

B Staple has been edged
into the glenoid neck

140

Discussion of Procedures

Recurrent anterior dislocation of the shoulder is a common problem, especially among athletes. Many procedures have been devised to address this condition, five of which have been presented. With the exception of the arthroscopic repair, all of those discussed have been in common use for many years. There are numerous studies available documenting the effectiveness of these procedures in preventing recurrent dislocation (Table 13–2). There is such a plethora of procedures, all reported to yield good results, that at least one author (37) has observed that the actual technique of the repair is not half so important as making the decision to do a repair.

Because all of the operations discussed appear to give excellent results in terms of preventing recurrent dislocations, recent evaluations have centered on functional results, such as preservation of power and especially range of motion. This is often critical to the athlete. Occasionally, the type of repair must be dictated by the pathology that is present, but often there are several types that may be equally effective. In this case, the nature of the sport, level of competition, and the athlete's ultimate goals within his or her sport must be considered and weighed against the limitations of each surgical procedure.

Both the Putti-Platt and the Magnuson-Stack procedures are technically easy and effective at controlling redislocation. However, both repairs functionally shorten the subscapularis tendon and significantly impair external rotation. For a football lineman, or an ice skater, this may have no significant effect on their ability to participate. Throwing athletes, on the other hand, depend upon external rotation of the shoulder in abduction to give the whipping power to their motion. A 20-degree loss of external rotation will end the career of a baseball pitcher. Therefore, these operations are probably not suitable for an athlete who wishes to continue a career in such a sport.

At the present there does not seem to be any truly satisfactory operation for the high-level throwing athlete. The Bristow procedure was originally popularized as a repair that would not limit external rotation and was therefore advocated for athletes. However, long-term studies by Hill (17) and May (27) make it clear that although the loss in external rotation may not be as great, there is still a definite restriction. In Hill's study this loss averaged 12.6 degrees, which was sufficient to prevent all but 15% of his throwing athletes to return to their preinjury level of performance. Similarly, although the Bankart repair appears to be very satisfactory in the general athletic population, only one-third of the throwers in the series of Rowe et al. (39) were able to return and pitch as hard or throw a football as far as they had been able before injury. It has been argued that at least a one-in-three chance is better than no chance at all, and therefore the Bankart repair should be the procedure of choice in throwing athletes; however, clearly a 33% success rate is not satisfactory. Therefore, we feel that although the patient has a predictable chance that his problem with recurrent shoulder dislocations can be successfully treated surgically, one must make it clear to a throwing athlete that a return to his previous level of performance is unlikely. With this in mind, the surgeon must individualize his choice of surgical procedure, taking into consideration the underlying pathology involved and the patient's goals and expectations. It is possible

Figure 13-16 One arm of the staple is inserted through the middle glenohumeral ligament tissue and in this case the proximal subscapularis tendon as well, and is ready to be driven into the anterior glenoid (**A**). Staple has been driven home (**B**).

Table 13–2 Incidence of Recurrence Following Various Reconstructions for Anterior Dislocations of the Shoulder

Procedure	Authors	Year	No. cases	Recurrence (%)
Putti-Platt	Adams	1948	37	5.4
	Brav	1955	41	7.3
	Jeffery	1959	34	3.0
	H. Osmond-Clarke	1965	140	1.4
	Truchly	1968	102	0
	Leach et al.	1981	78	1.2
			432 Total	3.0 Average
Magnuson-Stack	Giannestras	1948	31	6.4
and modified	Palumbo and Quirin	1950	13	0
Magnuson-Stack	Vare	1953	30	0
	Alldred	1958	10	0
	DePalma and Silberstein	1963	75	2.7
	Jens	1964	42	9.0
	Bryan et al.	1969	53	7.5
	Magnuson and Stack	1943	6	0
	MacAusland	1956	21	9.5
	Gartland and Dowling	1954	14	0
	Robertson	1954	14	0
	Karadimas et al.	1954	154	2.0
	Aamoth and O'Phelan	1980	40	2.5
	Hovelius et al.	1977	68	1.9
		1979	571 Total	4.1 Average
Bankart and modified	Adams	1948	18	5.5
Bankart	Townley	1950	26	0
	Rowe	1956	75	1.3
	Du Toit and Roux	1956	150	5.0
	Dickson and Devas	1957	50	4.0
	Boyd and Hunt	1965	49	4.1
	Rowe et al.	1978	145	2.5
			513 Total	3.3 Average
Bristow	Helfet	1958	30	3.0
	McMurray	1961	73	2.7
	May	1970	16	0
	Collins and Wilde	1973	50	0
	Hill et al.	1981	107	2.0
	Lombardo et al.	1976	51	2.0
	Nielsen et al.	1982	18	0
	Barrett et al.	1982	50	4.0
	MacKenzie	1980	16	0
	Hummel et al.	1982	81	0
	Hoveius	1983	111	6.0
	Allman	1974	50	0
	Sweeney et al.	1975	97	3.0
			750 Total	1.7 Average

[Reproduced with permission from C.A. Rockwood. In: C.A. Rockwood and D.P. Green (eds.) Fractures in Adults, pp. 722–985. J.B. Lippincott, Philadelphia, 1984 (21).]

that the arthroscopic staple capsulorrhaphy will become the procedure of choice in the throwing athlete. Intellectually, it would appear to offer the chance for the least loss of motion. However, no long-term follow-up is currently available on this procedure, and its effectiveness remains to be established. Future treatment appears to be moving toward less invasive ways of repairing anterior shoulder instability. Those attempting these new techniques should spend time benefiting from those who have been using them. There are numerous potential pitfalls and many new innovations coming. It will be another 5–10 years before arthroscopic repairs establish their place in treatment of anterior shoulder instability. In most cases the results from traditional methods are so predictable that these procedures remain the treatment of choice at the present time.

References

1. Adams JC. The humeral head defect in recurrent anterior dislocations of the shoulder. Br J Radiol 23:151–156, 1950
2. Bankart ASB. The pathology and treatment of recurrent dislocation of the shoulder joint. Br J Surg 26:23–29, 1939
3. Bost F, Inman V. The pathologic changes in recurrent dislocation of shoulder. A report of Bankart's operative procedure. J Bone Joint Surg [Am] 24:595–613, 1942
4. Brav EA. An evaluation of Putti-Platt reconstruction procedure for recurrent dislocation of the shoulder. J Bone Joint Surg [Am] 37:731–741, 1955
5. Broca A., Hartman H. Contribution a l'etude des luxations de l'epaule. Bull Soc Anat Paris 4:312–336, 1890
6. De Anguim C. Recurrent dislocation of the shoulder—roentgenographic study. J Bone Joint Surg [Am] 47:1085, 1965
7. De Palma AF, Silberstein CE. Results following a modified Magnusen procedure in recurrent dislocation of the shoulder. Surg Clin North Am 43:1651–1653, 1963
8. De Palma AF, Cooke AJ, Prabhakar M. The role of the subscapularis in recurrent anterior dislocations of the shoulder. Clin Orthop 54:35–49, 1967
9. De Palma AF. Surgery of the Shoulder, 3rd Ed, p. 474. JB Lippincott, Philadelphia, 1983
10. Du Toit GT, Roux D. Recurrent dislocation of the shoulder, A 24 year study of the Johannesburg Stapling Operation. J Bone Joint Surg [Am] 38:1–12, 1956
11. Eyre Brook AL. Recurrent dislocation of the shoulder. Lesions discovered in 17 cases: Surgery and intermediate report on results. J Bone Joint Surg [Br] 30:39–48, 1948
12. Flower WN. On pathologic changes produced in the shoulder joint by recurrent dislocation. Trans Path Soc London 12:179–200, 1861
13. Gianestras NJ. Magnusen-Stack procedure for recurrent dislocations of the shoulder. Surgery 23:794–800, 1948
14. Helfet AJ. Coracoid transplantation for recurring dislocations of the shoulder. J Bone Joint Surg [Br] 40:198–202, 1958
15. Hermodsson I. Rontgenologische Studien über die traumatischen und habituellen Schultergelenk-Verrenkungen nach varn und nach unten. Acta Radiol (Suppl) 20:1–173, 1934
16. Hill HA, Sachs MD. The grooved defect of the humeral head: a frequently unrecognized complication of dislocation of the shoulder joint. Radiology 35:690–700, 1940
17. Hill JA, et al. The modified Bristow-Helfet procedure for recurrent anterior shoulder subluxations and dislocations. Am J Sports Med 9:283–287, 1981
18. Hoppenfeld S, DeBoer P. Surgical Exposures in Orthopedics: The Anatomic Approach. JB Lippincott, Philadelphia, 1984
19. Hovelius L. Shoulder dislocation in Swedish ice hockey players. Am J Sports Med 6:373–377, 1978
20. Hovelius L. Incidence of shoulder dislocation in Sweden. Clin Orthop 166:127–131, 1982
21. Hovelius L, Thorling J, Fredin H. Recurrent anterior dislocation of the shoulder. J Bone Joint Surg [Am] 61:566–569, 1979
22. Jobe F, Jobe C. Painful athletic injuries of the shoulder. Clin Orthop 173:117–124, 1983
23. Joessel D. Ueber die Recidine der Humeras-Luxationen. Deutsche Zeitschrift Für Chirurgie 13:167–184, 1880
24. Johnson LL. Instrument Makar Video Digest. Instrument Makar, East Lansing, MI, June 1984
25. MacDonald FR. Intraarticular fractures in dislocations of the shoulder. Surg Clin North Am 43:1635–1645, 1963
26. Magnuson P, Stack J. Recurrent dislocation of the shoulder. JAMA 123:889–892, 1943
27. May VR. A modified Bristow operation for recurrent dislocation of the shoulder. J Bone Joint Surg [Am] 52:1010–1016, 1970

28. McLaughlin HL, Cavallaro WU. Primary anterior dislocation of the shoulder. Am J Surg 80:615–621, 1950

29. McLaughlin HL, MacLellan DI. Recurrent anterior dislocation: A comparative study. J Trauma 7:191–201, 1967

30. Miller LS, Donohue JR, Good RP, Staerk AV. The Magnuson-Stack procedure for treatment of recurrent glenohumeral dislocations. Am J Sports Med 12:133–137, 1984

31. Moseley HF. Recurrent Dislocation of the Shoulder. McGill University Press, Montreal, 1961

32. Moseley HF. The basic lesions of recurrent anterior dislocation. Surg Clin North Am 43:1631–1634, 1963

33. Osmond-Clarke, H. Habitual dislocation of the shoulder. J Bone Joint Surg [Br] 30:19–25, 1948

34. Palmer I, Widen A. The bone-block method for recurrent dislocation of the shoulder joint. J Bone Joint Surg [Br] 30:53–58, 1948

35. Perthes G. Uber Operationen bei habitueller Schulter Luxation Deutsch Ztschr. Chir 85:199–227, 1906

36. Pilz W. Zur Roentgenentersuchung der Habituellen Schulterverrenkung. Arch f klin Chir 135:1–22, 1925

37. Rockwood CA. Subluxations and dislocations about the shoulder. In: Rockwood CA, Green DP (eds). Fractures in adults, pp 722–985. JB Lippincott, Philadelphia, 1984

38. Rowe CR. Prognosis in dislocation of the shoulder. J Bone Joint Surg [Am] 38:957–977, 1956

39. Rowe CR, Patel D, Southmayd W. The Bankart procedure. J Bone Joint Surg [Am] 60:1–16, 1978

40. Schultze E. Die Habituellen Schulterluxationen. Arch f klin Chir 104:138–179, 1914

41. Simonet WT, Cofield RH. Prognosis in anterior shoulder dislocation. Am J Sports Med 12:19–23, 1984

42. Simonet WT, et al. Incidence of anterior shoulder dislocation in Olmsted County, Minnesota. Clin Orthop 186:186–190, 1984

43. Symeonides PP. The significance of the subscapularis muscle in the pathogenesis of recurrent anterior dislocation of the shoulder. J Bone Joint Surg [Br] 54:476–483, 1972

44. Townley CO. The capsular mechanism in recurrent dislocation of the shoulder. J Bone Joint Surg [Am] 32:370–380, 1950

45. Watson-Jones R. Fractures and Joint Injuries, 4th ed. Williams & Wilkins, Baltimore 1957

Index

Techniques in Orthopaedics
Editorial Board

Contents
Revision of Total Hip and Knee
Edited by Lawrence D. Dorr

Contents

Topics in Orthopaedic Trauma
Edited by Phillip G. Spiegel

Contents
Update in Arthroscopic Techniques
Edited by William A. Grana